DEMONS

DEMONS

Our changing attitudes to alcohol, tobacco, & drugs

VIRGINIA BERRIDGE

OXFORD
UNIVERSITY PRESS

OXFORD
UNIVERSITY PRESS

Great Clarendon Street, Oxford, OX2 6DP,
United Kingdom

Oxford University Press is a department of the University of Oxford.
It furthers the University's objective of excellence in research, scholarship,
and education by publishing worldwide. Oxford is a registered trade mark of
Oxford University Press in the UK and in certain other countries

Published in the United States of America by Oxford University Press
198 Madison Avenue, New York, NY 10016, United States of America

British Library Cataloguing in Publication Data
Data available

Library of Congress Control Number: 2013940971

ISBN 978–0–19–960498–2

Printed in Great Britain by
Clays Ltd, St Ives plc

ACKNOWLEDGEMENTS

This book is the product of many years' interest—initially in opium and other drugs in the nineteenth and twentieth centuries and subsequently in other substances, including alcohol and tobacco. My location as an historian in non-historical settings, starting with the Addiction Research Unit at the Institute of Psychiatry and currently at the London School of Hygiene and Tropical Medicine, have brought me into contact with non-historical frames of thought, which have greatly enriched the writing. The time spent as scientific secretary of a cross-research council and government department research initiative made me aware of policy and I have remained an interested participant observer in the field.

Many colleagues have influenced what is written here, but I am particularly grateful to Wayne Hall, whose sabbatical taken in the Centre for History in Public Health in 2012 came just at the right time; to Stuart Anderson for his helpful connections with historians of pharmacy in Europe; and to Jane Falconer from the LSHTM library for bringing me up to speed with search techniques. Other colleagues, among them Robin Room and Alex Mold, helped with references and advice. Alex also acted as reader of the semi final text and made helpful comments and suggestions. My role as leader of a work package on 'addiction through the ages', part of the EU's Framework 7 programme on addiction and lifestyles, helped to open my eyes to European perspectives in a field that is often dominated by the Anglo-American. My involvement in both historical and substance networks has been helpful. Here I should mention the Alcohol and Drugs History Society, the Society for the Study of Addiction and the International Society for the Study of Drug Policy. Many funders have supported work which feeds into the book, among them the Economic and Social Research Council, the

Joseph Rowntree Foundation, the Alcohol and Education Research Council (now Alcohol Research UK), and the Nuffield Trust (formerly the Nuffield Provincial Hospitals Trust). Particular thanks go to the Wellcome Trust, which supported my post at a crucial period and which has given invaluable support to the Centre for History in Public Health.

I have used the open access resources of the Wellcome library in the course of writing this book: the Centre's Tavistock Place location could not be better for visiting that Euston Road treasure trove. Senate House Library is also an invaluable local asset, both for books and for online journals.

I am grateful to my editors and to the team at Oxford University Press: Luciana O'Flaherty who originally suggested the idea of a book with a different title and framework; and in particular Latha Menon, whose astute advice on structure helped make sense of a host of potential avenues, and whose continuing hands-on involvement has improved the end product. Emma Marchant (now Ma) helped to nudge the text through and Sophie Basilevitch provided excellent support in picture research. As always, Ingrid James has been a great support in the Centre office; and my family and friends make sure there are plenty of things other than drugs to think about.

CONTENTS

LIST OF ILLUSTRATIONS

1
Introduction: Past and Present

Scientists writing in the *Lancet* in 2007 argued that there should be a rational scale for assessing the harms caused by 'drugs of potential misuse'. Drugs, as they pointed out, were regulated according to agreed classification systems. Yet there was no confidence that the classification systems adequately reflected the actual harms these drugs caused. The scientists, led by the ebullient psychopharmacologist Professor David Nutt, then a member of the government's Advisory Council on the Misuse of Drugs (ACMD) developed a nine-category matrix of harm. They also included five drugs of misuse which were legal—alcohol, khat, solvents, nitrites, and tobacco—and one, ketamine, which was classified later. Their ranking, not surprisingly, produced a different assessment of harm to that used by the regulatory systems currently in operation in Britain and internationally. Heroin was still at the top of the harm list, but they listed legal drugs like alcohol and tobacco way above substances such as cannabis, LSD, and Ecstasy, all classified more strictly under the British Misuse of Drugs Act. They concluded

> Our results...emphasize that the exclusion of alcohol and tobacco from the Misuse of Drugs Act is, from a scientific perspective, arbitrary. We saw no clear distinction between socially acceptable and illicit substances. The fact that the two most widely used legal drugs lie in the upper half of the ranking of harm is surely important information that should be taken account of in public debate on illegal drug use. Discussions based on

formal assessment of harm rather than on prejudice and assumptions might help society to engage in a more rational debate about the relative risks and harms of drugs.[1]

The uncompromising stance attracted widespread interest in the media. Leading scientists prepared to say that alcohol was more harmful than crack cocaine clearly invited a news story. Some experts criticized the basis on which the 'harms' had been calculated and argued that the evidence used was skewed in certain ways. The same group of scientists published a further paper in 2010 which attempted to deal

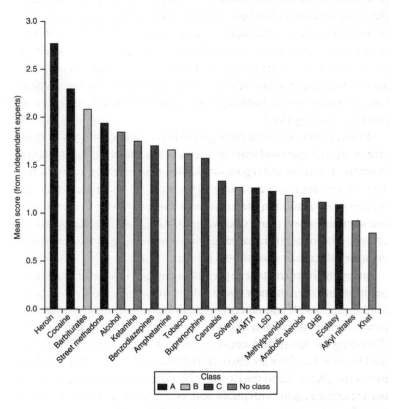

FIGURE 1 *Lancet* 2007 ranking of substance harms.

with the adverse comment. Basically, their aim was to criticize current systems of control, both for legal and for illegal drugs. The scientists' willingness to stride into the debate emphasized that society was going through a time of flux in relation to attitudes and practices surrounding the use of mind-altering substances. These are some of the questions which this book also addresses, but it starts from a different perspective. Its focus is on history and its argument is that history is central to an understanding of the positioning and response to substances. It does not state what should happen in the future, but looks back to the past, both recent and more distant. This approach allows us to identify the issues which have led these different substances to their current status in culture and in regulation in society. We can then ask: which way is society heading today so far as substance use is concerned—towards greater hedonism, or greater restriction? What brings change and why are national responses so different? Are attitudes to substances which have, in recent history, been separate—drugs, alcohol, and tobacco—moving closer together?

Demons aims to examine through the lens of history why these substances moved apart and whether they are now moving closer together in terms of cultures and regulation. Unlike many commentaries in the area, the text does not have a 'line' to promote. It looks at the historical process of separation in the nineteenth and early twentieth centuries and identifies a new phase of coming together from the late twentieth century. The focus is on analysing what is happening and may develop in future rather than what should happen.

Surveying the current scene presents a confused picture. Drinking to get drunk has been the new youth culture in the UK. Twenty-four-hour drinking is possible and supermarket drink discounts are controversial, now leading to discussion of government imposed minimum pricing. Illicit drug use has spread: cocaine is everywhere, often in association with alcohol. But there are also contradictory tendencies. The smoking ban in the UK has led to the closure of licensed premises. Cannabis has been restricted again, with public support. Abstinence from drink and from drugs has mainstream support in the USA and increasingly in the

UK. Illicit drug use is in decline. Meanwhile, some scientists and medical professionals call for 'drugs for all', a brave new world of cognition enhancers and designer drugs which can help everyone to be happy. They stress genetic factors and pathways in the brain. Happiness, or 'wellbeing' is the end point and licit and illicit drugs should be considered together in rational systems.

The aim of this book is to make an argument which is grounded in history, both in the deeper past and more recently. It will examine and analyse how the process of redefining substances has taken, and is taking place. How are substances defined and framed and how and why do definitions and responses change? What factors are involved? Does culture or does regulation have most impact? How do those two polarities interact? How are substances defined as presenting particular sets of problems and why do those definitions differ?

In bringing the substances together to ask these questions, I will contest two types of argument which have dominated in discussion.

One argument pays attention to the *properties* of the substance—drugs of various types, alcohol, or tobacco—and their range of harms. Drugs were made illegal, the argument goes, because they were dangerous. Such a particular substance-focused explanation has been around a long while but still needs unpicking. It lacks historical depth and fails to recognize the range of time-contingent factors which have brought the substances to the positions they occupy. It also separates the substances from each other.

The other argument is the more recent one. It recognizes the different historical trajectories the substances have taken. It argues that it is now time to throw out that baggage and to *classify the substances 'rationally'* according to actual harms. If tobacco or alcohol were to be discovered recently, so the argument goes, there is no way they would be legal substances now. This second argument implies that history can be dismissed. But it cannot. And the argument that the positioning of substances can be changed just like that is really part of the current story and the analysis of this book: it is part of the process in the here and now by which substances are being repositioned and recategorized.

I will argue that too much attention has been paid to the impact of systems of regulation in isolation or to tired catch-all explanations such as 'moral panic', still over-used to explain responses to drugs. We will look at particular factors which have impacted on responses to drugs:

- the role of the state;
- of vested and economic interests like the tobacco and alcohol industries (which also vary cross-nationally);
- activism;
- local and national tensions;
- differing professional interests; and also
- international interests, the role of international agencies and networks.

Culture is bound up in the process: in general, substances with widespread cultural legitimacy are not easily made the subject of stringent systems of control. For example, alcohol was not totally prohibited in the 1920s in the USA, and Gorbachev's anti-alcohol policies in the 1980s in Russia fell victim to widespread popular opposition. But increased regulation in turn impacts on culture and helps to change it; and that cultural change in turn opens the door for further regulation. It is an iterative process.

We have had clear examples of this with the opiates in the nineteenth and early twentieth centuries; and, more recently, with tobacco. Back in the 1950s, who would have thought that people would be banned from smoking in pubs and restaurants or in their offices? No politicians would have tangled with that issue: fifty years later they were prepared to. The smoking ban shows how the legislation was contested—but once in place, it has helped to define new cultural norms and further detached tobacco from cultural acceptability. It has also had an impact on attitudes to alcohol as well, as an unexpected side effect.

The argument thus has echoes of Malcolm Gladwell's famous *Tipping Point*—the process which turns an object from 'uncool' to 'cool', or the other way round. Although Gladwell was primarily concerned with what causes change, his was not an historically focused set of explanations but rather one leaning towards social psychology.[2] For substances, both regulation and culture and their interaction need to be built in. This is an historical process which is open ended and changing as we write and speak. Science itself with its proponents is a player in all of this. The changing concepts which are used to characterize the substances are outgrowths of a matrix of influences. These concepts are often seen as timeless and value free, as 'pure science'. The rise of interest in addiction to nicotine, for example, now so prominent in current debates, is not a belated recognition of an immutable scientific fact, but rather a concept that has suited changing scientific and policy interests to espouse, given the changing cultural and legal positioning of tobacco in society, as the book discusses in Chapter 10. The recent arrival of neuroscience on the substance agenda has been seen as 'pure science' even by some historians but, this book argues, its rise to significance is also rooted in specific policy agendas.

The repositioning of substances is a complex process. This book aims to make readers aware of the complexity, to make them realize that there is more to changing responses to, and positioning of, substances than just a simple realization of 'dangers' and 'harms'. Rationality in looking across the substances may now be on the agenda but we should also examine the roots of that current debate, its implications in the 'new genetics' and its dependence on the past. One side effect of the recent discussions has been that the 'legalization' versus 'prohibition' debate has become perhaps less dominant than it was. There is a dawning realization that systems of regulation and control have been very variable and are difficult to encompass under such 'catch-all' descriptions. If we look through the history of the last two centuries, and across different countries, a multiplicity of forms of regulation appear. These range from complete open availability; to controlled availability of various sorts, including licensing and government or other types of monopolies; prohibition; criminal and legal forms of control; medical controls; and public health responses through prevention and other forms of public health input. Even categorizing in this way does not fully encompass the forms of control; and many of those systems outlined here overlap with each other. One recent analysis of drug policy called the twentieth-century 'British system' of drug control one of prohibition.[3] But what the author was really characterizing was a system of controlled availability with medical controls through prescribing and the prescription pad. The doctor was the gateway to access for addicts and for other patients. The use of the term prohibition as a category often simply denotes a stance; it means any system of control with which an author does not agree.

This book aims to look at why certain substances are legal now and others are not in Western societies, taking the opiates primarily as examples for the 'illicit' branch, and alcohol and tobacco for the 'licit' route. The time frame and key issues are discussed over two broad periods: the nineteenth century through to the 1920s; and the 1950s to the near present. One can identify a broad trajectory whereby all these 'drugs' started with some form of availability in the nineteenth century, but by the early years of the twentieth century they had gone down rather different routes—legal for alcohol and tobacco, illegal for the opiates and associated drugs such as cocaine and cannabis. A renegotiation of boundaries had taken place in terms of regulation but also in the way in which the substances were categorized. For a 'drug' can also be both medicine and food; paradoxically, alcohol lost its status as a medicine by the early twentieth century, while opium (at least in the form of its alkaloids: morphine, codeine, and heroin) retained it. The early decades of the twentieth century were a key turning point for this overall process of separation, with the First World War important because of its impact on the different paths taken by drugs and alcohol.

But then the focus shifted. Another period of key change was the period after the Second World War. Tobacco came to the fore, gaining its status as a central problem for the revived postwar public health. 'Risk' was the category which exemplified new public health directions. It seems as if our substances, even the legal ones, had gone down very different paths. But even as they separated, there were elements of coming back together. Public health concepts began to be applied to drugs and alcohol, while increasingly tobacco and its active principle nicotine, began to be seen as a 'drug'. Ideas about 'addiction' and about harm reduction became the stuff of discussion across the substances. In some respects concepts changed places, with talk of tobacco 'addicts', but of drug 'users'. Medication and treatment as prevention has become a common tactic across the substances, with interventions varying from methadone to nicotine replacement therapy (NRT). Social movements have aided the reconceptualizations which have been played out on the international, even global, stage. Universalizing scientific concepts from epidemiology to brain science have played a key role in pulling the substances together. The final sections of the book will examine how some of those factors which had operated historically to delineate different paths have come into play in recent times to draw the substances closer together.

Let's begin by looking at the 'prehistory' of the substances before the nineteenth century. All had long histories which show similarities, with both social and medical usage entwined. Alcohol first. Beer has been said to be the first drink deliberately made by man.[4] It was brewed from fermented barley by the Bronze Age civilizations of Mesopotamia and Egypt in the third century BC. By the thirteenth century its central role in British diet and social life was recognized by a national Assize of Ale (1267) which established a maximum price per gallon according to a sliding scale of corn prices. According to Henry Jackson in 1758, 'Beer, commonly call'd Porter, is almost become the universal Cordial of the Populace', thus stressing popularity but also supposed health benefits. In the context of British culture, wine has held a more ambiguous place, with less general acceptability and consumption until recent times. But it, too, has a long history and viticulture began in the Aegean in the third millennium, with grape wine traded from Israel to Egypt.[5] Even in Britain, wine drinking began earlier than might have been expected, with the Domesday survey of 1086 identifying 130 English vineyards, 78 lay and 52 under church control. But wine drinking did not expand, even with the growth of wealth in the nineteenth century and the increased size of the middle classes. James Nicholls, in his history of alcohol, has shown how imbibing different substances, wine or beer, became identified with different styles of party politics in the late seventeenth century. The rise of gin just a few years later added spirit drinking to this combustible political mix.[6]

Tobacco, our other legal substance, was, as Jordan Goodman has pointed out, the first of the new 'exotica' to enter Europe as a result of the expansion of European interests overseas.[7] It took almost a century, from Columbus in 1492 to the publication in 1571 by Nicolas Monardes of his natural history of medicinal plants of the New World, for Europeans to take up the habit. By the early seventeenth century tobacco had become a global crop. In England, tobacco was a mass consumption commodity by around 1670 and possibly before that; enough tobacco was available for 25 per cent of the adult population to have at least one pipeful a day.[8] The Dutch were also avid tobacco consumers, and pipe production rocketed. Chewing tobacco, a custom observed in the Americas, was however, less congenial to European tastes. But there is evidence of an increasing proportion of people using snuff rather than tobacco in eighteenth-century Europe.

On the illicit side, 'drugs' have rather similar histories, dating back to ancient times. Opium, the product of the opium poppy, has been known in medicine for around 6,000 years, and was possibly the first drug used by early man. It had an early and honoured place in Greek, Roman, and Arabic medicine. References to the juice of the poppy appear in Assyrian medical tablets of the seventh century BC and in the Sumerian language around 4,000 BC the poppy is called the 'plant of joy'. In England, the drug had been used early on, chiefly for its narcotic properties. In the middle of the fourteenth century, John Arderne used salves and elixirs containing opium to procure sleep and even as a form of anaesthetic during operations. 'he schal slepe so that he schal fele no kuttyng'. The drug's soporific and narcotic qualities reappear in Chaucer's *Canterbury Tales* and also in Shakespeare, in particular in the famous passage from *Othello*:

Not poppy, nor mandragore,
Nor all the drowsy syrups of the world,
Shall ever medicine thee to that sweet sleep
Which thou ow'dst yesterday[9]

Cannabis too had an ancient history. The variety of names by which different parts of the plant are known—from hashish to marijuana—was in itself testimony to the drug's established place in the culture of many Eastern countries. Hashish was called esrat in Turkey, kif in Morocco, and madjun when it was made into a sweetmeat with butter, honey, nutmeg, and cloves. It had been known to the Chinese several thousand years before Christ and the Greeks and Romans had used it for both medical and social purposes. Cannabis was also known in Northern Europe before the nineteenth century. In 1689, for example, Dr Robert Hooke brought it to the attention of the Fellows of the Royal Society. Indian hemp, which 'seemeth to put a man into a dream' might, he thought, 'be of considerable use for lunatics'.[10]

The coca leaf and coca chewing had been known, like tobacco, since the discovery of the Americas. But unlike tobacco, its use as plant product did not translate into Europe. The drug had originally been regarded by the Incas as a symbol of divinity and hence became known originally in Europe through the medium of traveller's tales. Many descriptions were enthusiastic about the sustaining properties of the leaf. Abraham Cowley, an English physician and poet, celebrated the virtues of coca in his *Book of Plants* (1662).

Endowed with leaves of wondrous nourishment, whose juice sucked in, and lo the stomach taken long hunger and long labour can sustain. From which our faint and weary bodies find more succour, more they cheer the dropping mind, than can your Bacchus and your Ceres joined.[11]

What this brief survey has not explained is how these substances, initially grown in particular regions or localities, made the transition to substances whose use was spread worldwide. This was part of a process which the historian Alfred Crosby has called the 'Columbian exchange', whereby microorganisms confined to one part of the world translated across the Atlantic—in both ways. The exchange of diseases brought smallpox and measles into the New World, syphilis into the old, with consequences for both.[12] The American historian David Courtwright has applied this idea to the movement of drugs and other substances. 'The globalization of wine, spirits, tobacco, caffeine bearing plants, opiates, cannabis, coca, and other drugs...was a deliberate, profit driven process.'[13] He identifies what he calls a 'big three'—alcohol, tobacco, and caffeinated products—which were part of this 'psychoactive revolution'. The scale of their production and consumption and their integration into culture made them impervious to prohibition. A 'little three'—opium, cannabis, and coca—also made the transition, but were less integrated into culture than the other substances, eventually becoming the subject of prohibitions and restrictions. Courtwright also draws attention to substances which did not make the transition to globalization despite having attractive psychoactive effects and sanctioned cultural usage. One of his examples is khat, which has of course, recently begun to buck the trend. Khat is now flown into Heathrow airport every day to satisfy the tastes of the Somali population in London— although it has still not made the transition to widespread popular demand in the culture as a whole. When the Somali-born British Olympic runner Mo Farah gained his gold medal in the London Olympics in the summer of 2012, his brother, a farmer in Somaliland, delightedly told journalists that he would buy khat for his neighbours to celebrate. The book will discuss the current indeterminate status of the drug in Chapter 11.

This book starts with most of these substances comfortably translated into Western societies (cannabis and coca were the exceptions) in the nineteenth century. Why did they then take different paths? Some analysts have tried to formulate reasons why societies respond differently to different social issues. The American political scientist/ sociologist Constance Nathanson, for example, once compared smoking and gun control to see what had brought about different reactions in different countries. Some had more stringent control on tobacco than they did for guns. Yet the basic 'facts' about the issues were the same across those countries.[14] Why then did responses differ? Nathanson identified three factors: the role of the state—whether this was a country where there was a strong central state or not; the efforts of activist groups; and perceptions of risk. Nathanson was not looking at longer-term trends but more at the recent past of her topics. But her approach, moving away from a topic or substance-specific approach, makes a good start.

In the nineteenth century, the cultures of alcohol consumption, opiate use, and tobacco smoking were not that different and were widely embedded in social custom in the UK and also elsewhere. But over the next century and a half, they went their different ways. Why did they take these divergent paths? This book identifies a wider range of issues and the ways in which they impacted differentially on the substances. The argument is that economic and technical change associated with industrial societies interacted with the social movements characteristic of the time. Industrial interests were important. At the same time the professionalization of medicine and pharmacy, and the introduction of systems of medical discipline and control, led in some countries to increased state control, or at least the aspiration for such control. Public health also came into the equation. Public health concerns were part professionalization and part social concern so not totally altruistic. Fear was also a potent force. If the substance was associated with a feared or despised minority or section of the population, it was easier to take stringent action against it. Finally, the international and global scene has been a powerful agent and location of different control strategies. Such factors operated either to detach a substance from mainstream culture or to embed it more firmly in the period up to and including the First World War.

This is a complex process, so, to make the points clearer, I will take this analysis forward through a series of case studies on each issue, sometimes focusing on one substance and sometimes on another, depending on which is most significant. This is not a comprehensive history; the UK is the main focus with other cross-national comparisons, with Europe brought into the picture alongside the ever-dominant

US story. The text will show how the substances moved down separate paths. Then it will turn to show how they have been reconceptualized since the Second World War. In the late twentieth century and early twenty-first centuries there have been signs that all are now becoming 'drugs'. The matrix of factors which drew them apart in the early twentieth century seems to be operating to draw them closer together. I will conclude by looking at this more recent process, outlining ways in which the 'case study' issues have continued to operate.

2
Culture: Drugs for All

Thomas De Quincey first took opium in 1804. Plagued as he was with rheumatic pains in his head and face, a college friend recommended it.

> It was a Sunday afternoon, wet and cheerless: and a duller spectacle this earth of ours has not to show than a rainy Sunday in London. My road homewards lay through Oxford Street; and near the stately Pantheon (as Mr Wordsworth has obligingly called it) I saw a druggist's shop. The druggist, unconscious minister of celestial pleasures!—as if in sympathy with the rainy Sunday, looked dull and stupid, just as any mortal druggist might be expected to look on a Sunday: and when I asked for the tincture of opium, he gave it to me as any other man might do: and furthermore, out of my shilling, returned to me what seemed to be real copper halfpence, taken out of a real wooden drawer.[15]

The effect on him was far from dull.

> I took it—and in an hour, oh! heavens! What a revulsion! what an upheaving, from its lowest depths, of the inner spirit! What an apocalypse of the world within me! That my pains had vanished, was now a trifle in my eyes: this negative effect was swallowed up in the immensity of those positive effects which had opened before me—in the abyss of divine enjoyment thus suddenly revealed. Here was a panacea...for all human woes: here was the secret of happiness...happiness might now be bought for a penny, and carried in the waistcoat pocket: portable ecstasies might be corked up in a pint bottle; and peace of mind could be sent down in gallons by the mail coach.[16]

The poet's use of the drug as described here stressed its aid to expanding consciousness. This was a type of recreational use, which in the nineteenth century would have been called the 'luxurious' use of the drug. The place of what would later come to be called 'non-medical' use of opium in the genealogy of Romanticism in the nineteenth century has been discussed by a variety of biographers and literary critics.[17]

The memoir also gives a clue to different ways in which opium was used in nineteenth-century society. That De Quincey could go to a druggist and buy the drug over the counter tells us something significant. For this anecdote opens the door to a world of drug taking not connected to the expansion of consciousness, to literary or artistic usage, but rather to opium as part of everyday life, the type of product which anyone could buy.

This chapter looks at cultural acceptability. In the first half of the nineteenth century 'drugs', whether opium, alcohol, or tobacco, were widely available in society, culturally sanctioned, and acceptable. Our three sets of substances were all more or less tolerated socially, although with rumblings of concern, at least so far as opium and alcohol were concerned. In this discussion, the focus is initially on opium, because its cultural acceptability is more unusual when looked at from the vantage of the present. There is some reference to the parallel situations of alcohol and tobacco. This chapter examines how substances which later came to be considered separately both within society and in terms of regulation formed an overall culture of 'substance use' at the time.

England is the case study and opium use there was completely unrestricted before 1868 when the first Pharmacy Act became law. The London drug wholesaling markets had their cases of opium alongside other imported drugs and spices. Opium was imported from Turkey through normal channels of commerce as one more item of trade. The London based drug wholesaling houses had extensive lists of opium products, which predated the nineteenth century.[18]

Numerous opium preparations were available. There were opium pills, lozenges, powder of opium, opiate confection, opiate plaster, opium enema, and liniment. There was the famous tincture of opium, (opium dissolved in alcohol), known as laudanum and the camphorated tincture or paregoric. The dried capsules of the poppy were used, as were poppy fomentation, syrup of white poppies, and extract of poppy. Nationally famous and long established preparations such as Dover's Powder vied with a tranche of new commercial preparations from the mid nineteenth century—the chlorodynes, Collis Browne's, Towle's, and Freeman's. Childrens' opiates like Godfrey's Cordial and Dalby's Carminative were everyday purchases.There were local preparations such as Kendal Black Drop, known only because Coleridge used and wrote about it.

The Apothecaries Company had twenty-six opium preparations available in 1868, including its popular 'cholera number two' mixture. One wholesale druggist was selling poppy capsules at 1/10d a hundred, opiate plaster, Hemming's extract of opium and syrup of white poppies, Battley's Sedative solution, morphine acetate, and hydrochlorate, Turkey opium, as well as Black Drop and special Godfrey bottles (three dozen for ten shillings). Godfrey's cordial was an opium based patent medicine.[19] Local wholesalers, even at the end of the century, had extensive opium lists. W. Kemp and Son at Horncastle offered nine opium preparations in 1890. There were special quotations for twenty-eight pound and fifty-six pound lots of Turkish opium. There were even short-lived attempts to grow opium commercially in England—but the weather and the shortage of labour defeated these.

What was this extensive variety of opium-based preparations being used for? Medicine of course was one area. Medical practice relied extensively on opium at the time. The pharmacologist Jonathan Pereira noted in his textbook of materia medica in 1839 that the drug was used

> to mitigate pain, to allay spasm, to promote sleep, to check nervous restlessness, to produce perspiration, and to check profuse mucous discharges from the bronchial tubes and gastro-intestinal canal.[20]

It would almost be easier to list conditions which did not use opium than those where its use was central. For it was essentially a palliative.

There were few specific cures for diseases in the first half of the nine-teenth century, germ theory lay in the future, and many diseases remained to be medically defined. Opium provided pain relief and an intermission which might aid recovery. For cholera its use remained virtually unchallenged. In the 1849 cholera epidemic, the *Lancet*, reporting on the treatment of cholera in the London hospitals, commented 'This disease does not yield to the ordinary remedies to which common, and even severe autumnal diarrhoea yields, as chalk mixture, etc. Its best remedy is opium, given judiciously, but fearlessly.'

The author of the piece had been called at 3 a.m. on Saturday to a child on the Surrey side of the Thames, aged fourteen months.

> He was well at bedtime…at one a.m., the mother looked at the child, and found it awake, the bed soaked with gushes of *mere water* from the rectum, and the poor little fellow vomiting, every few minutes, pale fluid; his legs drawn up. He was ordered—Wine of opium, ten minims; sulphuric ether, half a drachm; cinnamon water, six drachms. Of this mixture one third was given every half hour, carefully watching, to pre-vent narcotism.
>
> He took all three doses of opium, the vomiting and purging ceased, he retained lime water and milk in his stomach, some reaction occurred, in a few hours he fell asleep, and awoke in the evening, well but weak.[21]

For insanity, too, it provided a more humane response than earlier methods which had used physical restraint. Dr John Connolly, one of the leading figures in the movement to establish different responses to insane people, recognized that it could act differently on different people.

> With some patients laudanum acts with certainty, and like a charm; others derive comfort for long periods from the acetate of morphia; to some the liquor opii sedatives is alone tolerable. Whatever sedative is employed, the dose should be large. Less than a grain of the acetate of morphia is productive of no good effect whatever; and laudanum requires to be given in doses of a drachm, or at least of forty or fifty drops. I am speaking of acute cases, for in those of longer continuance, use often makes much larger doses necessary.[22]

In one particular variant of insanity, delirium tremens, the drug was often used to sober the patient up. Thomas Jones, a coachman who drank extensively, was admitted to Kings College hospital in London in 1850, reported as seeing devils running about. His treatment was a diet of porter, beef tea, and brandy, with laudanum every three hours.[23]

Outside such medical practice, then available to only a very small minority of the population, lay widespread popular use of the drug. In Chapter 4 we will look at how our different drugs were sold and made available to the public. Opium was available through small general stores as well as the druggists mentioned by De Quincey. Corner stores were the mainstay of working-class districts and the shops were often kept by people little better off than the populations of the areas they served. In factory areas, the wives of factory workers would keep shops to help supplement the family income. Such shops were plentiful and the vendors were often ill educated. A business in Scarborough which had a day book with recipes used listed 'red oils for cattle', alongside an infants' preparation and one for 'coff drops', based on 'Loddanum, parreygorick' and other drugs.[24] Dispensing knowledge was picked up where the sellers could, assuming they were literate, which the Scarborough shopkeeper barely was. They relied on self-help books such as William Bateman's *Magnacopia*, published in 1839. Opium-based recipes for astringent balls, gout remedies, and corn plasters mingled with others for ink, cleaning grates, and making preserves. In the small corner shops, 'they put down their penny and get opium'. Vendors sometimes had their own specialities, especially in the 'children's draught' line of business.

Street markets also sold opium preparations. According to Samuel Flood, a surgeon in industrial Leeds in the 1840s, Saturday night purchases of pills and potions were a regular habit alongside buying meat and vegetables. He commented 'in the public market place...are to be seen...one stall for vegetables, another for meat, and a third for *pills!*'[25] Medical herbalists who were common and untrained midwives in working-class areas also had their own recipes. An untrained medical adviser to poor families would prescribe mixtures containing laudanum for diarrhoea and dysentery, widespread complaints because of poor sanitation and living conditions.

These opium preparations were developments of self-dosing before industrialization. Poppy-head tea had long been a regular remedy used by families in the country before they moved to the new industrial towns and cities. It was a remedy for fractious babies and also for adults. Laudanum was later the most popular form of opiate. Everyone would have it at home—it was the aspirin or paracetamol of its day. Twenty to twenty-five drops could be had for a penny. Working-class lives became very separate from those of the middle and upper classes, and few at that level realized the extent of use. It only emerged when special enquiries were made. One such was from a committee enquiring into the sale of poisons in the 1850s. Professor Arnold Taylor told the enquiry, 'in many large manufacturing towns...labouring men come to the extent of two or three hundred a day for opium'. Edward Hodgson, a pharmacist in the northern town of Stockton-on-Tees, decided to make a record of whom he served with opium in one summer month in 1857. Two hundred and ninety-two customers bought opium from him during that time. Hodgson was one of six qualified chemists in the area, so that presupposes that at least sixty people each day were buying opiates from these outlets (excluding others lower down the retail scale). This was the pattern outside industrial areas as well. The day-book of William Armitage, a 'chemist and grocer' in Thorne, a village near Doncaster, shows how normal sales were made. Between June and December 1850, he sold pennyworths of laudanum, two-pennyworth of paregoric to Mrs Coulam on 6 September, a mixed order of laudanum, acid drops on 10 July, with five pence left owing for opium by Stephen Webster; the entries show the acceptability of opiates as everyday purchases.

In one rural area, opium use was particularly noticeable. This was the low lying marshy Fenland area covering parts of Lincolnshire, Cambridgeshire, Huntingdon, and Norfolk. The area was remote and attempts at drainage uncompleted, and the Fens were subject to frequent flooding. In the first half of the nineteenth century, the fenland remained an unhealthy, marshy area, and those who lived there were prone to the 'ague', 'painful rheumatisms', and neuralgia. It had been known for some decades that these conditions led to a noticeably higher use of opium in the area. One analysis published in 1862 commented that more opium was sold in Cambridgeshire, Lincolnshire, and Manchester than in other parts of the country. Poppy-head tea was common, as in other country areas. In the nineteenth century, more commercial opium prepations were used. Greater awareness of the custom and investigation of it took place through the numerous social surveys and public health investigations of the time. The high death rate in rural Lincolnshire drew particular attention to it in the 1860s and Dr Henry Julian Hunter was sent there to investigate on behalf of the Chief Medical Officer of the day, Sir John Simon, who was medical officer to the Privy Council.

He wrote

> A man in South Lincolnshire complained that his wife had spent a hundred pounds in opium since he married. A man may be seen occasionally asleep in a field leaning on his hoe. He starts when approached and works vigorously for a while. A man who is setting about a hard job takes his pill as a preliminary, and many never take their beer without dropping a piece of opium into it. To meet the popular taste, but to the extreme inconvenience of strangers, narcotic agents are put into the beer by the brewers or sellers.

In the 1880s, Dr Rayleigh Vicars, who practised in Boston in Lincolnshire, was perplexed by the symptoms displayed by one of his patients. One of her friends soon set him right. 'Lor, Sir, she has had a shilling's worth of laudanum since yesterday morning.' Dr Harper, working at the dispensary in Holbeach, was surprised at the longevity of the opium consumers he saw. Fifteen who came to the dispensary had an average age of seventy-six years, although all were taking over a quarter of an ounce of the drug each week.

Opium taking reached its peak in the Isle of Ely. It was a well-known centre of opium distribution and the surrounding towns and villages, March, Doddington, Chatteris, and Whittlesey also had high opium consumption. In 1894, Thomas Stiles, a druggist who was then in his nineties, remembered the quantities he had dealt in.

[D]aily I supplied a vast number with either opium or laudanum...The amount of opium consumed in the commencement of the present century in this form was enormous, and it is surprising the quantity of laudanum which was taken with impunity, after being habituated to its use.

Opium was to be bought in the county town of Cambridge on market day. The Christian Socialist writer Charles Kingsley used this to make an East Anglian encounter in his novel *Alton Locke*

'Yow goo into druggist's shop o' market day, into Cambridge, and you'll see the little boxes, dozens and dozens, a 'ready on the counter; and never a ven-man's wife goo by, but what calls in for her pennord o'elevation to last her out the week. Oh! ho! ho! Well, it keeps women-folk quiet, it do; and it's mortal good agin ago pains.'
  'But what is it?'
  'Opium, bor' alive, opium!'

Opiate use on the Fens was culturally accepted and sanctioned in a way which recalls the cultural acceptability of alcohol or tobacco at the same time. The majority of the population and local shopkeepers clearly accepted its use as quite normal, even well into the 1870s and 1880s. In Boston, Dr Rayleigh Vicars struggled against community support for the habit in order to try to bring a medical imprint to the situation. 'The neighbours', he reported, 'indulge in the same lethal habit, and encourage the fatal termination by good naturedly lending their own private store of laudanum.' Buying opium was a child's errand, just like other small purchases. In Croyland in the Fens, one had the 'daily duty...to go every morning for a shillings worth of opium, or, as it was nicknamed, "stuff"'.

The overall lack of concern was demonstrated by an encounter in a chemist's shop in Wisbech in 1871. The writer reported how he

went into a chemist's shop, laid a penny on the counter. The chemist said 'The best?' I nodded. He gave me a pill box and took up the penny,

and so the purchase was completed without my having uttered a sylla-
ble. You offer money, and get opium as a matter of course. This may
show how familiar the custom is.[26]

It was the dosing of children with opiates which first drew the attention
of public health interests and this was a more general matter of concern
in the public health movement in the nineteenth century. The Registrar
General's reports fuelled this concern.These showed that the highest
proportion of opium poisoning deaths occurred among young children, especially babies less than a year old. Between 1863 and 1867, 235
babies under one had died, and fifty six children aged between one and
four. Three hundred and forty children and adults over five had died.
On average during those years, 20.5 poisoning deaths from opium per
million population had occurred in the under fives; the rate in the over
thirty-fives was 7.8 per million. Soothing syrups were popular purchases from chemists and from corner shops. Godfrey's Cordial, Dalby's Carminative, Daffy's Elixir, Atkinson's Infants' Preservative, Mrs
Winslow's Soothing Syrup, and Street's Infant Quietness were among
the many preparations, national and local, which crowded the market.
A series of public health investigations into factory life from the 1830s
onward drew particular attention to the connection between womens'
work and 'infant doping'. Evidence was collected from the industrial
towns and cities and the availability of mortality figures through the
newly established (1830s) General Register Office, showed the high
rates of infant mortality in some of those towns. The voluntary public
health movement brought its influence to bear. The Manchester and
Salford Sanitary Association was one such. It held public lectures in the
1850s and 1860s on 'The Injurious influence of certain narcotics upon
human life, both infant and adult'. The Association expressed its anxiety about infant doping as one of the examples of working-class mis-
management of their children.

> Few but those who have been much among the poor, know how
> fearfully mismanaged their little ones are—how the infant shares his
> mother's dram and all her food, from red herring to cucumber—
> how he takes medicine sufficient homeopathically to treat the whole

community—and how finally, an incautiously large dose of laudanum wraps him in the sleep that knows no waking.

Such examples of concern could be multiplied and carried with them
certain assumptions—that the mother's absence at work was the root
cause and that 'ignorant nurses' were also at fault. Such stereotypes did
not always represent reality and many mothers did not work full-time.
Opium was to some extent a palliative for the gastrointestinal complaints which in conditions of poor housing and sanitation caused
most infant illness and death. Nevertheless, it did have some role to
play in an imperfect system of infant management.

Occasionally, too, beliefs in the positive power of the drug for children creep through the torrents of criticism. The popular belief in the
power of opium as a restorative was reflected in terms like 'cordial' and
'preservative'. Preparations like Godfrey's were thought to be 'strength-
ening' and good to use for a sickly baby. In one parliamentary enquiry,
we find the testimony of Mary Colton, a twenty-year-old lace runner in
Nottingham, who had been advised how to care for her illegitimate
child by women in her community.

> She could not afford to pay for the nursing of the child, and so gave it
> Godfrey's to keep it quiet, that she might not be interrupted at the lace
> place; she gradually increased the quantity by a drop or two at a time
> until it reached a teaspoonful; when the infant was four months old it
> was so 'wankle' and thin that folks persuaded her to give it laudanum to
> bring it on, as it did other children.

The campaign had a well-founded target but it was also myopic, for it
ignored the extent of use outside these circles of workers. Opium was
well used in the nurseries of the well to do, as 'home companion' advice
books demonstrate. Prescription books with their opiate-based preparations show that opium solutions were widely dispensed for middle-
class infants.

In general, apart from such 'doping' use, working people and those
higher in social status, were relying on the drug for a whole range of
minor complaints. They were a cure-all for conditions, some trivial,

some serious, for which little other attention was available. The drug was for instance widely used for sleeplessness. The number of opiate-based cough remedies, 'chest tonics', and rheumatic and diarrhoea pills in chemists' recipe books gives an indication of the range of conditions where opium would be a standard home remedy. These uses paralleled those in orthodox medical practice. Self-medication with opium prob-ably encompassed a broader range of complaints than those dealt with by trained medicine. The connection of opium and drink was one such, although as we saw earlier, opiates did come into use in medicine for the treatment of delirium tremens. In everyday life, it was used to coun-teract the effects of too much drink, as an informal means of 'sobering up'. In Liverpool in the 1850s opium was sold by publicans during the cholera season and in the fruit season in the summer, 'It is the custom for the publicans to keep a supply of laudanum to add to the brandy...' This in fact appears to have been a widespread means—which also emerges through the Fenland accounts—of controlling and counter-acting excessive drinking, as an informal means of sobering up.[27]

Victorian society mostly saw drug use as 'normal', more than a cen-tury before the 'normalization' of drug use became a subject of public discussion in the 1980s. Drugs were in use in the 1850s at the popula-tion level, with higher rates in some areas than in others. The advent of registration of births and deaths in the 1830s enabled some idea of over-all patterns of use to be gained. Child mortality from opiates was high in some areas. Deaths from opium were high (140 died from narcotic poisoning in 1868) and there was a high level of accidental overdose. But whether the figures were rising or not is open to doubt. The rate in 1840 of five per million population for narcotic poisoning deaths had risen to six per million by the 1860s—not a steep increase, considering the first figure was probably an underestimate. Import statistics show that home consumption was rising, although not as swiftly as contem-poraries thought.

What concerned Victorian society initially was not 'addiction'—that concept was in the future and is discussed later on in Chapter 4. It was a quality issue—the variability of the drug as sold to consumers. The high accidental death rate was due to the lack of standardization of what people bought over the counter. In 1863, 106 of the 126 opium deaths were accidental. The deaths or near misses involving public figures drew attention to the problem. The Earl of Westmoreland was handed a phial of laudanum by his manservant in mistake for another medicine, and was only saved by prompt action with the stomach pump. Accidental overdoses were a fact of everyday life. When Mr Story took over a shop in Guisborough in 1858, with an existing stock of groceries, draperies, and drugs, he felt he was not experienced in selling drugs. But the vendor pressed him to take the whole stock. Fanny Wilkinson, a local servant, sent for powdered rhubarb. It was not surprising that Story confused the jar marked 'Pulv.opii Turc. Opt.' (Turkish opium) with Turkish rhubarb. Fanny died after taking a teaspoonful of powdered opium; Mr Story had to stand trial for manslaughter. Such cases could be multiplied time and again. Dealing with an opium overdose was commonplace and appeared as a standard section in most books of domestic medicine, self-help medical advice. Buchan's *Domestic Medicine*, published in the early nineteenth century, and which thereafter went through numerous editions, gave full instruction for blistering plasters on the arms and legs, stimulating medicines, the use of 'strong vomits', and drinking warm water with oil to bring up the poison. Professor Robert Christison, an eminent pharmacologist, wrote of what he called the 'peculiar sopor' caused by an opium overdose. The person affected had an expression of 'deep and perfect repose'. He could always be roused, although with difficulty, but as soon as the stimulation was removed, this lethargy would return and death often followed.

Christison was also involved in investigating the quality of drugs sold; for a major concern in the first half of the nineteenth century was the adulteration of all sorts of food and drugs. He bought laudanum from seventeen different shops, fourteen in Edinburgh and three in a Scottish country town. These gave wildly varying percentages of morphia, one of the active principles of the drug. Further evidence of the lack of quality control was publicized in the *Lancet*, then a radical campaigning journal under the editorship of Thomas Wakley. The journal published an 'Analytical Sanitary Commission' in 1853–4, which revealed the details of adulteration of food and drink, and also drugs such as opium. Nineteen out of the twenty-three samples of gum opium purchased were found to be impure, with the most common additives being poppy capsules and wheat flour. But not until later in the century, in the 1870s, did the sale of adulterated drugs become punishable.

Habitual use, what we would now call addiction, caused less concern. One can speculate as to why this was so. It was possible, indeed probable, that quite large numbers of the population were what we would now call 'addicted' or 'dependent' on opium. But this reliance was not always obvious. Supplies were available and it was only if they were suddenly interrupted that the situation became plain. The surveys and the anthropological accounts of the late twentieth century were far in the future. Patterns of use appear haphazardly, and the survey which Christison and a surgeon, G. R. Mart, carried out in the 1830s, was very unusual for the time. This recorded twenty opium eaters, thirteen women, of whom seven could be called working class, and seven males, two of whom were workers. Their habit was known and acknowledged, so that fact alone made them out of the ordinary. Most addiction went unremarked. In the Lancashire cotton famine of the 1860s, when supplies of cotton to the northern cotton towns were interrupted because of the American Civil War, unemployment and destitution was rife and the purchase even of pennyworths of opium was difficult. Robert Harvey was at that time an assistant to the house surgeon at Stockport Infirmary. At the end of his career he had become the Inspector General of civil hospitals in Bengal and reflected on his earlier experience while giving evidence to the Royal Commission on Opium in the 1890s.

> Many applications were made at the infirmary for supplies of opium, the applicants being then too poor to buy it ... 'I was much struck...' he recalled, 'by the fact that the use of the drug was much more common than I had any idea of, and that habitual consumers of ten to fifteen

grains a day seemed none the worse for it; and would never have been expected of using it.'

Doctors who worked closely with the poor in other areas also glimpsed the extent of habituation. Dr Frances Anstie, the editor of *The Practitioner*, wrote about the prevalence of opium taking among poor people in London.

> It has frequently happened to me to find out, from the chance of a patient being brought under my notice in the wards of a hospital that such a patient was a regular consumer, perhaps, of a drachm of laudanum, from that to two or three drachms per diem, the same doses have been used for years without any variation.

His comments on this discovery were realistic. The consumers were 'persons who would never think of narcotizing themselves, any more than they would be getting drunk; but who simply desire a relief from the pains of fatigue endured by an ill-fed, ill-housed body, and a harassed mind'.

In such a situation, where the drug was freely available with, in the first half of the century, and even after that, minimal controls, the type of distinction between what was medical and what was non-medical use was more blurred than it became later on. In some areas such as the Fens, where usage was investigated in some detail, there was a recognition that consumers were taking the drug for part medical, part what we would now call recreational use. The writer Thomas Hood on a visit to Norfolk, was surprised to find out about opium eating in the Fens. '[T]he Fen people in the dreary, foggy, cloggy, boggy wastes of Cambridge and Lincolnshire had flown to the drug for the sake of the magnificent *scenery* ...'. Dr Rayleigh Vicars, who had grown accustomed to the unusual habits of his patients, also recognized this to be the case. His patients' 'colourless lives are temporarily brightened by the passing dreamland vision afforded them by the baneful poppy'. The lives of middle-class consumers, it should be remembered, were less subject to investigation. The liberal politician and prime minister, William Gladstone, took opium in a cup of coffee

before big speeches in the House of Commons, as did William Wilberforce, the reformer of the slave trade. Wilberforce had first been prescribed the drug for colitis in the 1780s and, in 1818, thirty years after
his first prescription, was still taking the same dose, a four-grain pill
three times a day. Lord Carrington commented of him some years
after that, 'it is extraordinary that his health was restored by that
which to all appearances would be ruined by it, namely the constant
use of opium in large quantities'. Wilberforce himself remained stubbornly resistant to dropping his opium, maintaining that the pains of
'growling guts' were more intolerable than his dependence on opium.
Opium was simply a part of life for many consumers, neither exclusively medical nor entirely social.

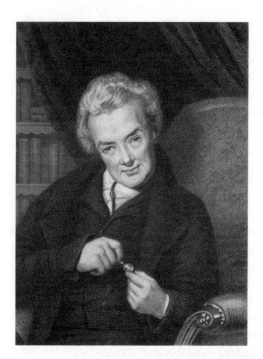

FIGURE 2 William Wilberforce, opium addict.

This, then, was the overall picture of British drug consumers in the nineteenth century. Drug use was common at all levels of society and was largely unconnected with medical practice before the arrival of the alkaloids of opium such as morphine (of which more later). This may not have been a universal model, even in European and North American countries. In the United States, it has been argued that 'addiction' (not use) was the outgrowth of medical prescription throughout the nineteenth century. Non-medical use there was mainly in the form of opium smoking. What happened in the States, so it appears, was a move away from iatrogenic (medical) addiction and a descent down the social scale, with a greater role for underworld consumers by the end of the nineteenth century. Such a picture does not correspond at all with the British case and even the type of medically induced addiction seems to have been different, as we will see in Chapter 8. But it is difficult to make comparisons. The historian David Courtwright, who has looked at the US situation, has focused his research primarily on what were termed 'addicts' rather than 'users' or 'consumers'.[28] He comments that the administration of opium and morphine by physicians was the leading cause of addiction in the nineteenth century. The data he utilizes comprises some pharmacists' records as well as those of doctors; he also uses import figures and formally issued medical prescriptions. In the British pattern of use outlined above, the prescription had little importance until the twentieth century, until after the advent of National Health Insurance. The terminology of addiction comes later in the British context; the extent of opium use in the general population via pharmacists seems to have been greater, with access from different sources of supply. The 'underworld' connection which Courtwright emphasizes has little parallel in the UK and even by the time of the First World War, the UK drug 'scene' was very small. Pharmacists did sell opiates over the counter in the USA as well but we know less about those general patterns of consumption in the US population.[29]

Other drugs which have acquired illegal status since the nineteenth century, primarily cannabis and cocaine, were much less central to Victorian society, and one cannot talk about a general culture of use.

Cannabis, known through travellers' tales of the Far East, was brought into the country by Dr William O'Shaughnessy, an Edinburgh educated Irishman. While out in India he first encountered the use of cannabis. His paper 'On the preparations of the Indian hemp, or gunjah (cannabis indica); their effects on the animal system in health, and their utility in the treatment of tetanus and other convulsive diseases' was published in 1842 in the *Transactions of the Medical and Physical Society of Calcutta*. O'Shaughnessy recommended that the preparation, both extract and tincture, should be used by medical men, and the pharmacist Peter Squire of Oxford Street was responsible for converting the resin into extract and distributing it to large numbers of the medical profession. But it was used infrequently in medical practice because of its uncertainty of action. O'Shaughnessy's advocacy of the drug's use for dysmenorrhoea and his attendance on Queen Victoria during childbirth led to the later widely repeated assertion that the Queen herself had used cannabis. This was a useful debating point for cannabis reformers in the 1990s but it appears to have little foundation in fact. Nevertheless the myth has continued to be circulated.[30] (It was galling for the author of this book to be told recently that her work had informed this conclusion—when the exact opposite was the case, and I had tried to debunk the myth.) In one area only—the treatment of insanity and of opium eating—did cannabis gain temporary popularity, ironically given its later denigration as a cause rather than a cure for mental illness. But of popular use on the model of opium there was none in the nineteenth century.

Coca, the leaves of the coca plant, had a similar limited role. Dr Paolo Mantegazza,who had practised medicine in Peru, published a work in Italian in the 1850s on his return to Europe and recommended the drug for a range of illnesses including toothache, digestive disorders, and 'neurasthenia'. Cocaine, the alkaloid, was in the process of being isolated. But it was the properties of the coca leaf which initially attracted most attention, with a number of doctors investigating them. There followed a period in the 1870s when 'lay' experimentation really took off. In 1876, the American pedestrian, Weston, used the coca leaf in walking trials in London. His conclusion was that the drug did not help maintain physical endurance. But others, including medical men, were enthusiastic about its potential use. Foremost among them was Sir Robert Christison, the Edinburgh pharmacologist who had been the investigator of opium in the 1820s. Now he became an advocate of the benefits of coca chewing. He made two 'walking trials' with coca leaves in 1870 and 1875. He was able to walk fifteen miles without fatigue and two ascents of Ben Vorlich in the Highlands were exceptional for a man of his age.

> My companions…were provided with an excellent luncheon…but I contented myself with chewing two thirds of one drachm of cuca leaves…I went down the long descent with an ease like that which I used to enjoy in my mountainous rambles in my youth. At the bottom, I was neither weary, nor hungry, nor thirsty, and felt as if I could easily walk home four miles.

Other medics were keen to promote its use for what might now be considered non-medical purposes. It was a cure for bashfulness, and helped in steadying the aim while out shooting. 'Filling my flask with the coca tincture, instead of with brandy…down went the birds right and left'.

Later it was used in patent medicines and coca wines; in 1894, there were at least seven firms producing coca wines for the domestic market.

Alcohol's cultural acceptability is better known. However, here too, certain misconceptions have crept into general discourse, as we will see. There is no doubt that heavy drinking and the consumption of large amounts of alcohol, especially by men, was seen as normal and even beneficial well into the nineteenth century. The *Gentleman's Magazine* in the eighteenth century recorded eighty-seven ways of saying someone was drunk. These ranged from the rather genteel 'sipping the spirit of Adonis' to the vulgar 'stripping me naked'. Hard drinking was notable at all levels of society. It was as acceptable for the local squire to fall dead drunk under the table after a night's drinking as it was for heavy labour to be leavened by periods of heavy drinking. Drink was embedded in all aspects of life and the rites of passage, christening, weddings, and funerals, were normally occasions for heavy communal drinking. During times of public celebration, ale and wine would be distributed to the common people. At Newcastle upon Tyne a fountain was constructed in the market place for George III's coronation, 'the conduit running wine all the time for the populace'.[31] Alcohol consumption and work were not seen as incompatible and periods of heavy labour would be alleviated by alcohol. In the eighteenth century, drink was built into the fabric of social life—it played a part in nearly every public and private ceremony, commercial bargain, and craft ritual.[32] Alcohol fulfilled many functions, even triggering carnivalesque behaviour in which the norms of everyday life were inverted. The poet and politician Samuel Bamford recalled his youth in early nineteenth-century Middleton in Lancashire, where on Easter Monday companies of young men in grotesque dress would stagger from house to house receiving gifts of money and ale, while 'men thronged the ale houses and there was much folly intemperance and quarrelling amidst the prevailing good humour'. On the following day a young fellow who had become so intoxicated as to be incapable, would be selected as mock mayor for the next year.[33]

But such vignettes of excess also mask a period of changing consumption from the eighteenth century into the mid nineteenth. The seventeenth and eighteenth centuries were the centuries when Europe had taken to 'soft drugs', including tea, coffee, and chocolate. From 1850 to the late nineteenth century there was a large increase in consumption; the consumption of beer, wine, and spirits all peaked around 1875. The consumption of tea also grew. These were trends which were associated with rising living standards.

Within the overall trends, different groups in Great Britain had very different drinking patterns. People in the countryside drank less than those in the towns and cities. Some groups were teetotal. It is not particularly helpful to talk of a 'British attitude to drinking', as there were large geographical variations in alcohol consumption. Across the UK, urban dwellers tended to consume more alcohol than their rural counterparts, and areas dominated by trades like mining and dock work also recorded higher levels. In 1900 the average per capita expenditure on alcoholic drink was estimated to be £4 10s 4d a year; the average dock worker was thought to spend 8s 4½d on drink every week…nearly five times as much as the average figure for the country.[34] In Nottingham, known for its hard drinking later in the twentieth century, the inns and public houses flourished because workers migrated from the rural areas to work in the town over the course of the eighteenth and nineteenth centuries. Pubs became social centres for the lower classes but their activities were often regarded as problematic. Trade and political groups were prohibited from licensed premises by Parliament in 1799 because of fears generated by the French Revolution. After relaxation of the laws however, trade union activities resumed in pubs. Branches often associated themselves with particular houses in the city. Shoemakers met at the Butchers' Arms, lace makers and printers met at the Durham Ox and framework knitters at the Dove and Rainbow, Seven Stars, and King George on Horseback.[35] So, although Britain was a 'hard drinking society' for much of the nineteenth century, there were peaks and troughs; this was not a timeless and universal aspect of the British character. Alcohol, like opium, also had its medical uses and these became the subject of agitations by medical temperance supporters later in the nineteenth century.

Smoking too had spread in Europe since its introduction in the sixteenth century. In England, tobacco had become a mass consumption commodity by the late seventeenth century at least. Enough tobacco was available for at least 25 per cent of the population to have a pipeful once a day.[36] And pipes it was at this stage. Until the invention of the cigarette for mass production in the second half of the nineteenth century, the clay pipe was a major means whereby tobacco was consumed. Cigars also spread among middle-class consumers and more widely in Southern European countries. British consumers turned to snuff from the late eighteenth century but not to chewing tobacco. Like opium, tobacco also had its medical uses and Goodman has noted that, like that drug, the boundaries between medical and non-medical (recreational) usage, are difficult to draw at this time.[37]

Britain entered the nineteenth century with more than half the tobacco market represented by snuff, but this proportion declined quickly. The pipe returned to the British tobacco scene and by the middle of the century, 60 per cent of British consumption was pipe tobacco. Pipes too changed during the century as more became manufactured of briar rather than clay. But clay pipe smoking remained common among working-class consumers. The habit was seen as essential for them to perform their everyday work. Publicans gave away pipes free and the association between drinking and smoking was close. In Wilkie Collins' novel *The Moonstone* (which also has an opium theme, for Collins was a laudanum user), on both occasions on which the character Gabriel Betteridge takes visitors to Cobb Hole, a small country cottage, 'good Mrs Yolland performed a social ceremony strictly reserved for strangers of distinction. She put a bottle of Dutch gin and a couple of clean pipes on the table, and opened the conversation by saying, "What news from London, Sir?" '[38] Like alcohol consumption, and that of opium, too, there were regional and local patterns of consumption with different tobaccos available for different tastes.

The century also saw the gradual social acceptance of cigar smoking, helped by support from Prince Albert, Queen Victoria's consort, an enthusiastic cigar smoker. Initial prejudice against aristocratic cigar smokers (women disliked the smell it left on the furniture and drapes) gave way to dislike of 'swells' who smoked cigars in the street. By the middle of the century cheaper cigars were more widely available and began to appear more widely in the novels of Dickens, Thackeray, and Trollope. Historian Matthew Hilton has stated that in the second half of the nineteenth century 'smoking was celebrated as the embodiment of the individuality of the bourgeois gentlemanly amateur'. Devotees collected the props of smoking culture, including clay pipes, briar pipes, pipe cleaners, matches, cigar holders, cigar cases, snuff boxes, and pipe racks.[39]

This chapter has shown how the substances were all more or less integrated into Victorian society. Tobacco, alcohol, and opiates were in common use, although in different ways and for different purposes. But they began to follow very different regulatory and cultural routes by the early twentieth century. Those paths were set at two stages: in the period around and just after the First World War, and again in the 1950s after the Second World War, when a further shift, focused in particular on tobacco, took place. The next chapters will examine the factors which impacted on changing culture and regulation: activism; professional, scientific, and technical interests; industry; international and global concerns; fear; against the backdrop of the changing role of the state and governments. All these operated to differentiate the substances from each other. We will begin by looking at the role of social movements and what would now be called activism: temperance is the first example.

3
Social Movements: Temperance

Joseph Livesey, a Preston weaver, had founded a temperance group within the Sunday school he ran for adults; many young men who attended signed the pledge of moderation in drinking. He felt that the alcohol in wine and beer was the same as that in spirits and equally harmful. So in 1832 he took the step which marked the birth of the British temperance movement.

> On Thursday, August 23rd 1832, John King was passing my shop in Church Street and I invited him in, and after discussing this question, upon which we both agreed, I asked him if he would sign a pledge of *total* abstinence, to which he consented. I then went to the desk and wrote one out...He came up to the desk and I said, 'Thee sign it first.' He did so and I signed after him...In the course of a few days notice of a special meeting was given, to be held in the Temperance Hall (the Cockpit), the following Saturday night, September 1st, at which this subject was warmly discussed...At the close of the meeting I remember well a group of us gathering together, still further debating the matter, which ended in *seven* persons signing a new pledge.

The pledge provided the founding charter of the temperance movement.

> We agree to abstain from all liquors of an intoxicating quality, whether ale, porter, wine or ardent spirits, except as medicine—John Gratrix, Edward Dickinson, John Brodbelt, John Smith, Joseph Livesey, David Anderton, John King.[40]

Only Livesey and King made much of a further contribution to the movement, but the 'seven men of Preston' assumed iconic status in later histories of temperance. A decisive change had taken place from the movement's initial focus on moderation and opposition to spirit drinking, but not to wine and beer, to opposition to all types of drink. That stance was to have significant consequences for society in the nineteenth and early twentieth centuries and also for the position of drinking and its regulation.

This chapter begins the consideration, in turn, of factors which have impacted differentially on alcohol, drugs, and tobacco. Each will be illustrated by means of a case study. Social movements, or the more restrictive term, pressure groups, can be major catalysts for policy and also for cultural change. In present-day society, we are used to the activities of campaigning groups across a range of issues. In the nineteenth century, such activity was a new development in the UK, which is where the case study is located. Movements like the one for the abolition of slavery, or for the abolition of the Corn Laws, represented something different in society. They brought together the organized efforts of men (usually so at this stage) to try to achieve changes in social attitudes but also in legislation. Temperance was part of that change in Victorian industrializing society. It affected culture, but also developed a political dimension, which began to draw upon the extended role of the state in the last decades of the nineteenth century.

It may seem a surprising and sudden change to be reading about a social movement focused on restriction, even prohibition, when the previous chapter has delineated the 'drink and drugs' culture of nineteenth-century society. The roots of temperance lay in wider changes in Victorian society. The historian Roy Porter drew attention to the emergence of philanthropic lobbies, fired by Evangelicism, and given over to rescuing drunkards.[41] Support for temperance also came crucially from self-respecting working men for whom it was a badge of 'respectability', that crucial concept for the upper levels of the Victorian working class. There were both moral and economic arguments against drink, in terms of its impact on social mores and the way in which it could aid the exploitation of workers, as in the custom of paying wages in pubs. Temperance reformers were accustomed to draw up an annual 'National Drink Bill' which drew up in economic terms the costs of alcohol and its misuse.

Temperance in Britain went through four major phases in its heyday of the nineteenth century. In the 1830s, it was a movement with clergymen and upper-class reformers leading a mainly middle-class membership. The focus was on the consumption of spirits, not wine or beer. Then the movement broadened to become a working-class one, and it became 'teetotal', aiming at total abstinence, as we have seen with the seven men of Preston. It was a vehicle for the self-improving upper levels of the working class, the 'labour aristocracy' for whom it provided a means of self-organization and a programme to aim at after the demise of the working-class political movement of Chartism. The movement also had support from Quaker and nonconformist business interests, and, later in the century, from the churches. The initial tactic was what was called 'moral suasion', that is, converting the individual who took the pledge, as the Preston men had, agreeing not to drink at all. American influence on the movement was important, in particular the passing of the Maine Law in 1846, which inspired British temperance supporters who wanted to bring prohibition into being. The British organization, the United Kingdom Alliance, was founded in 1853 to emulate the American example. From the 1870s onward, political tactics came to the fore and the movement aimed to infiltrate the Liberal Party as the likely vehicle of licensing reform. The aim was the so-called Permissive Bill, which would have allowed local preferences to decide what the drink situation should be in a particular neighbourhood. Voters would have to vote for or against the 'local veto' or local prohibition. The high point of this tactic was in the 1890s when the policy was central to the Liberals' Newcastle political programme. The nineteenth-century history of temperance showed how the focus of a social movement could change from the initial stress on individual responsibility to reliance on the role of the state.

So temperance had its influence in two overlapping worlds which are crucial to the positioning of substances—culture and policy. Let's look at its cultural impact first. The 1830 Sale of Beer Act gave a kick start to the early temperance movement's change of focus to total abstinence. The sale of beer, but not wines and spirits, was removed from control by licensing justices. Anyone could sell beer on payment of a two guinea fee. It was a free market solution which had an immediate impact. Over 24,000 licences were taken out in the first six months after the Act was passed and 21,000 over the following eight years. The Act coincided with a period of rural unrest and rioting, and an enquiry into this blamed it for a great increase in intemperance among the lower orders. The Act's existence gave a fillip to the growth of a movement which wanted total abstinence, although not all opposed free trade initially.

The teetotal movement had its initial strength in the north and among 'respectable' working men. Temperance advocates acted as 'missionaries' for the cause and a culture of temperance grew up. Thomas Whittaker, one of the Preston pioneers, gave a description of his activities during a visit to London in 1837 which gives a sense of the drive and enthusiasm.

> In London we are going on gloriously…During the last week I have held nine meetings and distributed 2,000 tracts; and large as London is I hope before long there will not be a soul in it who has not heard of teetotalism…On Saturday morning, I distributed 400 tracts on the Margate steamer; and in the afternoon, accompanied by several friends, went to Greenwich. On our way in the steam boat we preached up abstinence and the consequence was no intoxicating liquors could be sold, although they cried out 'Brown stout, ale and porter'. We held the first teetotal meeting ever held in Greenwich Park, and a good one it was. Returning home, I distributed tracts and gave admonitions at the dram shops.[42]

For those who joined the movement, there was a set of organizations inculcating sobriety and abstinence which in turn influenced a wider number in the general population. The doyen of temperance historians, Brian Harrison, attempted an estimate of how many actual temperance supporters there were. Here he drew a distinction between people who were actively involved and the wider circle who were influenced by temperance ideas.

> The general impression conveyed is that by the 1860s there existed an influential and literate minority in the country of 'opinion makers', numbering well under 100,000 teetotallers. The efforts of this minority affected the personal habits of at least a million adult teetotallers, and probably influenced the conduct of many others who did not join teetotal organizations.[43]

Temperance societies produced newspapers and tracts in their hundreds of thousands. There was a huge range of temperance literature. *A Dog's Protest Against Intemperance* in 1885, sang the praises of a drunkard's black dog, Keeper, who put his tail between his legs and trotted home when his master went into a pub. *Temperance in the Hay and Harvest Field* in the 1890s urged the end to free beer in the harvest field. *Tippling and Temperance* was a treatise of anti-drink sentences all beginning with the letter 't'. The novel *Danesbury House* by Mrs Henry Wood won a prize from the Scottish Temperance League in 1860 and was still in print at the end of the century. The story showed how drink could ravage a family. The misfortunes of the Danesbury family, owners of an engineering business, began when the baby William Danesbury was nearly poisoned by his drunken nurse. His mother, called home to nurse him, was killed in a carriage accident caused by a drunken turnpike keeper. Soon a new wife arrived, who pressed wine upon her stepchildren and children. The two older ones, Arthur and Isobel, refused out of loyalty to their teetotal mother's memory. William took an occasional glass while Mrs Danesbury's own children, Lionel and Robert, drank eagerly. The results were predictable. Arthur and Isobel did well as adults; William only narrowly escaped a drunkard's grave, Lionel died raving from delirium tremens, and Robert killed himself. Eventually Arthur opened a 'coffee public house' and made the village 'dry'.

Quakers became significant supporters of temperance and the Friends Temperance Union was established in 1850. This, like other societies, undertook widespread educational work often aimed at young children. Politicians such as the Liberal John Bright learnt their speaking trade through early involvement with temperance societies, in Bright's case, the Rochdale Juvenile temperance band.

The public meeting was central to reform campaigns and mass movements of the time. It was a way of demonstrating to government the power of the movement and also of attracting support. It was a form of recreation for working men, 'high mindedness and sheer good fun'.[44] Some of the accounts of teetotal meetings, especially in the early days, read like an entertainment, almost like music hall turns would be later on. The good temperance speaker would have the rapport with his audience and the showmanship of a professional working-class entertainer. The United Kingdom Alliance, a prohibition organization founded in the 1850s, used public meetings more than any other technique. As early as 1855, more than 500 Alliance meetings were held throughout the year in England, Wales, Scotland, and Ireland. By 1877, there were over 2,000 and by 1888, 4,000 with an attendance of over a million.[45] Some speakers had a standard patter which mixed humour with exhortation of the audience.

One of the most famous speeches was Joseph Livesey's 'Malt Lecture', which converted several people who later became prominent temperance reformers. 'Ladies and Gentlemen', he began, 'the greatness of a country consists not so much in its population, its wealth, or even in its general intelligence, as in its virtue'. Intemperance was costing the country £100 million a year. Why did people drink? From self-interest; from appetite; from fashion; from ignorance; from the 'great delusion' that alcohol was nourishing; and from 'deep depravity' because many, knowing the dangers of alcohol, continued to drink. To disprove ideas about nutrition Livesey entered into public demonstrations of the composition of alcohol, which greatly impressed his audience. He ignited the spirits obtained from evaporating a quart of ale and proved 'to the surprise and conviction of many who saw it' that it contained the same intoxicating ingredients as spirits. Livesey's lecture was franchised to other temperance speakers. 'I find that the exhibition has a theatrical effect upon meetings' said a teetotaller who performed the lecture in Wales.[46] Meetings were the location for what Harrison calls a 'peculiar form of secularized conversion experience';[47] this was the conversion to temperance and the taking of the pledge. This, too,

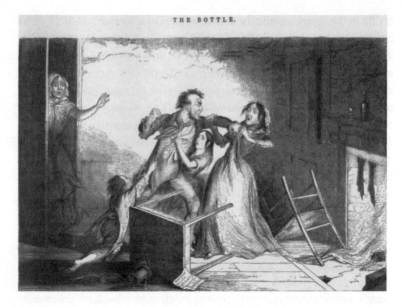

FIGURE 3 Cruikshanks 'The Bottle'.

was a theatrical experience and the temperance meetings paraded reformed drunkards to public gaze. All had a story of personal degradation and then redemption. Pictorial representations of the drunkard's career, such as Cruikshank's' *The Bottle*, which showed an inevitable progression in the other direction, from respectability to disgrace and poverty, were very popular.

In addition to the adult culture of temperance, there were several hundred thousand child teetotallers in the Band of Hope. Founded in 1847, membership was open to all children under 16, based on the simple pledge, 'I do agree that I will not use intoxicating liquors as a beverage.' In Leeds the Band was divided into sixteen districts and within a few months 4,000 children had been enrolled. In 1852, 6,000 children crowded into Exeter Hall in the Strand in London for a meeting. Thousands of children could not gain entry and the press of numbers stopped traffic in the Strand, while those inside the Hall adopted a formal presentation to the ten year old Prince of Wales.[48] By 1874, there were at least 5,500 Bands of Hope in the UK, with 800, 000 members, by 1889 the totals had risen to 16,000 societies and two million members, one in every four of the eligible age groups, and by 1897 to more than 3 million members.[49] Some Bands nested within existing Sunday schools, while other provided recreation and opportunities not available elsewhere. A specimen programme for Bands of Hope drawn up about 1881 suggested a variety of amusements for those attending, from a 'scriptural bee' to lessons in making temperance drinks. The first temperance song was written in the 1840s and its first verse went as follows:

> Come, all ye children, sing a song, join with us heart and hand
> Come make our little party strong, a happy temperance band.
> We cannot sing of many things, for we are young we know,
> But we have signed the temperance pledge a short time ago.[50]

Temperance has sometimes been criticized, either as a diversion from the real aims of working-class politics, in particular getting the vote; or as simply a way of imposing middle-class culture and manners on the working class, as something which 'civilized' them and drew them away from radical thoughts. But this was not the reality of the temperance culture. It was attractive to a particular type of Victorian working man (and later woman), a craft unionist, attracted by thrift, self-respecting and interested in religious matters. The reformer Josephine Butler, who campaigned in the 1870s and 1880s against the Contagious Diseases Acts, which penalized prostitutes but not the men who infected them, characterized them vividly.

> [T]he temperance men almost always lead in this matter—abstainers, steady men, to a great extent members of chapels and churches, and many of them are men who have been engaged in the anti-slavery movement and the abolition of the corn-law movement. They are the leaders in good social movements, men who have had to do with political reforms in times past, and who have taken up our cause. They may not be the majority, but they are men of the most weight and zeal in their

towns, and who have a considerable acquaintance with life, and large
provincial experience, and they gather round them all the decent men in
the place; when they start a movement they get all the rest to follow; and
properly so, because they are men of character.[51]

This comment tells us something about the support for temperance,
the particular brand too of temperance, nonconformity and provincial
vigour which marked Victorian life at this time.[52] Butler emphasized
the role of men in temperance but the movement was also notable for
the way in which women across the classes came together in association. Small female temperance groups came later than the male ones—
in the 1870s. The British Women's Temperance Association came into
being in 1876, influenced by American example. By 1892, led by the
redoubtable Lady Henry Somerset, it had nearly 600 branches and
45,000 members. Temperance was one of the first organized activities
in which women found a role in public life.

All this tells about the cultural change to which a social movement
can contribute. Certainly temperance supporters were always in a
minority, numerically speaking, but their influence was writ large.
They helped to rewrite the terms of the debate and indeed to initiate a
debate in a way which would not have been considered before. The
combination of association and abstinence was a powerful one. Change
in drinking habits was much to the fore by the 1870s, in part through
temperance promoted initiatives such as water drinking, the consumption of cordials, and the establishment of eating houses outside the pub.
Other developments, for example, the rise in working-class living
standards, which brought a move away from drink, had less to do with
temperance.[53] Temperance was a powerful influence—among others—
in helping to form a mass culture not founded on hard drinking.

Culture was one level where temperance had a profound influence.
But increasingly the movement also looked to the state to provide
solutions. From the 1850s, when the role of government was expanding
in other areas, public health for example, temperance supporters
looked to obtain solutions from government. The formation of the
Manchester-based United Kingdom Alliance (UKA) in 1853 brought

prohibition on to the agenda, inspired by the prohibition-based Maine Law (1846). The UKA believed that drink 'was a problem which required specifically public and political, rather than private and personal reforms'.[54] Faith in moral suasion was waning and there was an appetite for a more political approach. They argued that, as advocates of prohibition, they were also agents of liberation. They aimed to free consumers from the tyranny of drink, and also of the drink trade. An obvious counter to this was that prohibition itself would be a dictatorial solution. The answer was in the tactic of the local veto. Ratepayers in a particular area would be given the right to vote to go dry; a two-thirds majority would be needed. A bill for the local veto, the Permissive Prohibition Bill, was introduced into the Commons in 1864 and thereafter annually, with the MP Sir Wilfred Lawson as its champion.

For much of the next few years, the debate was dominated by what to do about licensing and the public house, and the connection with local government. Out of these electoral battles came the polarization of parties and electorates. Temperance reform became associated with the Liberal Party while the drink trade became associated with the Conservatives. Within the Liberal Party, the radical Liberal caucus organization, particularly strong in northern cities, saw local option and the local veto as a way of asserting their overall demands for the mobilization of the will of the people 'from below'. So the tactic of prohibition gained power through its association with these wider political objectives. The high point came in 1893 when the Liberal leader Harcourt was willing to introduce a bill which all the UKA wanted and which also denied publicans the right to financial compensation when they lost their businesses. But the Local Veto Bill never reached a second reading in 1895 and the Liberals fell from power, a fall which was widely interpreted as signifying public opposition to the policy of local veto. With hindsight, the defeat was more significant than it appeared to be at the time. It marked the end of the UKA as a significant force in Liberalism at the national level. Drink still continued to be a high-level policy issue in the first decade of the twentieth century. The defeat by the Lords of the 1908 Licensing Bill, which would have

accelerated and expanded reduction of licences, restricted compensation, and allowed for local referenda on the local veto, meant that the
issue became part of constitutional struggles over democracy. John
Greenaway in his study of licensing in this period explains the dominance of drink as a political issue between 1904 and 1908 by changes in
the composition of the parties themselves, in particular the dominance
of nonconformist Liberals in the Liberal Party. Drink also fitted into the
great issues of the day—the protection of property, the threat of 'social-
istic' legislation, and the rights of the people. Lloyd George used drink
cleverly as a means of arousing working-class support, with the brewers and the landed classes as easy targets.[55]

Drink was thus a useful party political issue, rather than a temperance
one. In fact, temperance as a social movement was in decline before the
First World War. There was no longer unanimity about what its main aim
should be. Back in the 1870s, Joseph Chamberlain, as Mayor of Birming-
ham, had promoted a different form of temperance solution called the
Gothenburg System. This Swedish port, much of interest to drink
reformers, had set up a trust company in 1875 run by unpaid directors.
This ran the local pubs—not to make a profit, but in order to invest the
returns into the town treasury and the local agricultural society. The aim
was to discourage drinking through higher prices, and shorter hours,
with pubs closing at 7 or 8 p.m. Managers could keep profits from food
but not from drink or from serving more than one drink per person.
Chamberlain, who had introduced 'gas and water socialism' to Birming-
ham in the form of municipal ownership of these utilities, also planned
to have 'beer and spirit socialism'. But he had been defeated in part by the
determination of prohibitionists to keep to their objective as the only
possible aim. In the early 1900s, aims within temperance became more
fragmented. In part this was because of the spread of different political
ideologies and discussion of the role which poverty played in drink consumption. The temperance argument had been that poverty was caused
by drink. In the 1900s reformers such as Joseph Rowntree began to look
at drink in a different way and to argue that licensing reform needed to be
part of a more general programme of social reform.

Rowntree and Sherwell's *The Temperance Problem and Social Reform*, which was published in 1899, was notable for the way in which it drew in examples from a range of countries to make its case. It argued that excessive drink consumption continued to be a problem but saw this in a different context to the prohibitionists. The dullness and monotony of working-class life was in part to blame, but also the capacity of the Trade, which could influence both national governments and local municipal life. The solution, so they argued, was to take the trade interest out of the sale of alcohol. Sherwell had visited the USA and Scandinavian countries in the course of his researches, and was convinced by the contrast between the shortcomings of the local veto in the USA and, by contrast, the operation of regulated management in Sweden and Norway. The first step in the UK could be the local authorities given the power to transfer a monopoly of the retail trade to specially formed 'disinterested management' companies, or even to local councils themselves. The profits would be handed to a central state-run authority which would hand profits back to localities in proportion to population and not to profits earned.

The issue of how to deal with drink thus divided the temperance movement before the First World War and beyond. Many temperance reformers were more interested in a moderate form of reform and some found a home in the Church of England Temperance Society. Although municipal or trust ownership never became official public policy, the 'trust' form of 'disinterested management' did spread at the local level. The most successful trust set up was not part of temperance. In 1901 Earl Grey began a campaign to raise the tone and restore country pubs. Several county trusts were formed, the most successful being the Hertfordshire Trust which took over The Waggon and Horses at St Albans. Within twelve months its takings from non-alcoholic drinks were nearly 70 per cent of its turnover. In 1919, this Trust expanded and became a public company, Trust Houses Ltd, controlling a hundred inns and hotels, the ancestor of the later commercial operation, the Trust House Forte chain.[56,57] These tactics have seen a revival more recently in the form of 'safer drinking practices' at the local level based on cooperation between local councils and publicans.

We can leave temperance as a social movement with a political pro-gramme in the decade before the First World War. What it had actually achieved at the cultural level is difficult to disentangle from a host of other changes taking place at the same time. Drink consumption began to decline in the mid 1870s. Some of this can be ascribed to the 'temper-ance effect' but working people also had access to holidays, leisure time pursuits not based on the pub-football and the music hall for example. Even rising living standards in these years and greater disposable income did not lead to rising levels of drink consumption. The temperance cul-ture itself had begun to feel 'old fashioned' even before the war and this was even more the case afterwards. Temperance reformers retreated within their own organizations rather than reaching out to a wider sym-pathetic audience. Politically, the movement had achieved something and we will discuss the particular case of the impact on women and children in Chapter 5. But it had not achieved prohibition or the power of the local veto. Alcohol remained set within the magistrate-run licens-ing system and drink as a party policy issue was in decline before 1914. Although licences were reduced in some areas, no overall prohibition or disinterested system of municipal liquor control came into being.

This chapter has used British temperance as its main case study to demonstrate how a social movement can help position a substance in a particular way at a particular point in time. Temperance did not oper-ate in the same way, or achieve the same outcomes, in all the nations which had strong movements. The great exemplar of a temperance movement which did ultimately achieve its aim, of prohibition, was that of the United States. What were the differences between temper-ance in the UK and in the USA? Some of the overall story in the USA is familiar from the British one. The movement began in the USA as in the UK as an anti-spirits one with support initially from economic entre-preneurs who wanted a more disciplined work force. By 1833 there were more than 6,000 societies and a million members pledged to total abstinence from the use of spirits.

In the 1840s it became more of a working-class organization, as the newly founded Washingtonian societies focused on working-class drunkards. After the Maine Law the aim became prohibition through an alliance of evangelicals, wealthy entrepreneurs, and respectable middle and lower-middle-class people united against the threat of pauperism and crime. Prohibition was achieved in thirteen states, a success which had no parallel in the UK. [58] Temperance and prohibition declined by the 1860s but then revived again from the 1890s with the establishment of the Women's Christian Temperance Union (WCTU) and the effective pressure group, the Anti-Saloon League (ASL), of great significance in piloting prohibition through the war.

So some elements of the story were the same—the move from anti-spirits to all drink and to prohibition; the widening basis of support from 'opinion formers' to the respectable working class. Some of the arguments made about liberty, in terms of liberation from the tyranny of drink, were also similar. The importance of temperance as a womens' movement was the case in both countries and in fact, there was much cross fertilization between the two. Frances Willard, the leader of the WCTU, spent time in the UK and Lady Henry Somerset and other British womens' temperance leaders visited the States and were much influenced by the model of abstinence promoted there. But there were clear differences in the sphere of religious enthusiasm. The evangelical equivalents of English dissent in the USA had no established church or hereditary aristocracy blocking their way. Ian Tyrrell has pointed out it was therefore relatively easy, by comparison to English temperance, for these US reformers to channel their views into socially dominant positions. The legislative victories for prohibition at the local level in the USA had no parallel in the UK. [59]

The timing and political ties of temperance in the two countries were also different. The British movement, despite its apparent importance in the pre-war Liberal government, was spent as a political force before the war. The American, by contrast, was on the way up. The Anti-Saloon League, by comparison with, for example, the United Kingdom Alliance, had no fixed political affiliations, but offered its impressive electoral machine to any politician who would support its anti-drink agenda. Prohibition was achieved in a significant number of US states, albeit temporarily, whereas in Britain the local veto was achieved for Scotland in 1913, the only country where it was still a living issue. The social basis and class structure of support was also different. As US historian Harry Levine puts it,

> The prohibition crusade was justified in terms of the needs of a new, complex, heterogenous, class stratified, industrial efficiency-oriented society of the twentieth century. The new prohibition ideology stressed the need to eliminate two particularly nefarious institutions: the liquor industry which was pictured as an enormously powerful and corrupt force; and the saloon, especially the urban, working class and immigrant drinking place.[60]

The new prohibition grew out of an alliance between the old middle class of small businessmen and the new middle class of professionals and technical experts, as well as representatives of the big corporations-all sharing a need to find ways of maintaining social, political, and economic order. The tactics of the ASL, and support from the Protestant churches joined with support from wealthy business men as the dominant deciding force. Big business saw great advantages in prohibition, in a way different to Britain, where the main business supporters came from nonconformist or Quaker backgrounds and the industry had its alliance with the Conservative Party.

Further comparison could draw out the differences in working-class culture between the two countries (temperance in the USA always accommodated working and lower-middle-class membership, rather than class specific organizations as in the UK); or the development of rival attractions; of the absence in the USA of welfare reforms and legislation providing holidays with pay. Political scientists like to use the concept of what they call 'path dependency', that is the trajectory of social or welfare policies in particular countries is to some extent predetermined by the prehistory of concepts, institutions, and their interaction. Britain and the USA show us how social movements can have similar aims but achieve very different outcomes in different countries with different structures and traditions.

Taking a wider international perspective shows further divergence. For temperance was a significant social movement in a particular set of geographical areas—in Northern Europe and North America. It was not important in Southern European countries, which developed very different responses to drinking and to alcohol. Even within Scandinavian countries, which are often lumped together as being 'anti-drink', there were clear differences. The historian Sidsel Eriksen has argued that the Swedes were most influenced by Anglo-American traditions and the Danes by German and that this made a difference to the success of temperance in the two societies.[61, 62]

So temperance as a social movement had a significant impact on attitudes and practices surrounding alcohol, although that impact varied crossnationally. What about our other substances? Here we can see that social movements and pressure groups were much less important, at least initially. Although there was some concern about the use of opium and of tobacco, there was no mass movement in opposition. The anti-opium movement in Britain had little of a working-class component and came into existence later than temperance, in the 1870s. The Anglo-Oriental Society for the Suppression of the Opium Trade (the Anglo-Oriental was later dropped) was founded in 1874. It owed its origin to the efforts of a group of Quaker anti-opium campaigners and to the unwavering support of the Pease family of Darlington, who were also Quakers. The Society initially ran a competition and prizes were offered for essays on the topic of *British Opium Policy and its Results to India and China*. Storrs Turner, an ex-missionary who was the first secretary of the Society won, and the book was published in 1876. This was the focus of the Society—not the situation in Britain, but in the Far East. Its main demands were for the abolition of the government monopoly of opium in India and the withdrawal of unfair pressure on the Chinese government to admit Indian opium. Support for the Society came from Quakers with the addition of some Church of England and Evangelical support—Lord Shaftesbury became its president in 1880. Motions for the withdrawal of the government of India from the opium trade regularly came before parliament and were regularly lost.

Opium was declining as a proportion of Indian government revenue from the 1880s and the Society's impact in Britain was limited. The anti-opium movement never achieved any broadly based provincial lobbying strength on the model of temperance. The height of its influence came in the early 1880s when it led calls for the ratification of the 1876 Chefoo Convention. The convention dealt with internal duties which could be imposed by the Chinese government and it allowed them to increase. In 1880, election year, the Society's election address gave commercial and moral arguments for ending the trade. A memorial signed by 360 members of the Society and other members of the public urging extinction of the trade and 'the duty of this country to withdraw all encouragement from the growth of the poppy in India, except for strictly medicinal purposes, and to support the Chinese government in its efforts to suppress the traffic' was presented to Prime Minister Gladstone in 1882. In 1882–3, there were 180 meetings on the opium trade, three times as many as in the previous year. The convention was ratified and thereafter support again waned until the 1900s. As with temperance, differences of opinion over strategy came into play. Some thought China should be the main focus, others thought India. In 1888 another anti-opium society came into being: the Christian Union for the Severance of the Connection of the British Empire with the Opium Traffic. Missionary influence was strong and it published its own journal *National Righteousness*. There was also a Women's Anti-Opium Urgency League and an Anti-Opium Urgency committee.

As with temperance, the anti-opium cause had high hopes of the Liberal victory of 1892. But anti-opium MPs were outmanoeuvred. A Royal Commission on Opium was appointed; its report in 1895 was regarded as a whitewash, although in some respects it simply acknowledged the reality of opium use in India.

> Opium is extensively used for non-medical and quasi medical purposes, in some cases with benefit, and for the most part without injurious consequences. The non-medical uses are so interwoven with the medical uses that it would not be practicable to draw a distinction between them in the distribution and sale of the drug.[63]

The anti-opiumists were as much prolific producers of tracts and pamphlets as the temperance movement. The SSOT had its own journal *The*

Friend of China, published at variable intervals. Most of the content dealt with China and India, although British example was occasionally drawn upon. De Quincey or Coleridge could illustrate opium eating. The Fens showed how opium could be used to treat malaria. Regulation in the two countries was also compared. The anti-opiumists made great play of the different legal frameworks for the availability and sale of opium. A children's story by Dr Emily Headland, *The Lady Britannia, Her Children, Her Step Children and Her Neighbours* pointed to the contrast. Lady Britannia, a 'loving mother', found that many of her children had taken a fancy to opium. But she took pains that they could not obtain it that easily, as it had to be labelled 'poison'. But with her step children it was different.

> They had been badly brought up before she took them in hand; she now sends them tutors and Governors…and is in many respects a model step-mother…It certainly is a strange thing, if she had any love for them, that she should let them buy this opium to their hearts content.[64]

Britain was not at all the focus of anti-opiumism, although attitudes developed from the Far Eastern case seeped over into British discussion— for example, that there was a clear distinction between medical and non-medical use; or that moderation in use was impossible. So the agitation, albeit limited in its successes, was preparing the ground for a different and more restrictive outlook on opium use. It was also, as we will see in Chapter 7, through its focus on the Far East rather than on Britain, paving the way for a significant divergence between alcohol and tobacco on the one hand and drugs on the other.

What about anti-tobacco agitation? The British Anti-Tobacco Society was formed in 1853. Of the initial 146 promoters, 38 were active scientists, the remainder moralists, evangelicals and social critics. Its secretary, Thomas Reynolds, was at times its only campaigner.[65] Later organizations included the Manchester and Salford Anti-Tobacco Society which became the North of England Anti-Tobacco Society and then, in the 1890s the British Anti-Tobacco and Anti-Narcotic League. Again there was a strong nonconformist element and support from manufacturers. Some temperance reformers were also anti-tobacco, but it was not until the anti-tobacco rhetoric became associated with fears about national decline in the late 1890s and early twentieth century that it achieved anything at all significant, as we will see in Chapter 5.[66]

We have looked mainly at temperance. That cause illustrates the importance of the great campaigning movement—but also its limitations. Social movements by themselves cannot determine greater restriction or freedom. But teetotalism's belief in total social transformation together with its mass membership, temperance as a 'way of life' as well as increasingly, a political strategy, had a profound effect. It did not achieve the aim of prohibition, for the cultural change which it also encompassed was accompanied by wider shifts in British social life, in particular among working people. But its influence can be seen in the fact that drink consumption did not rise as living standards did. People earned more and had more leisure time but chose not to spend it on drink. The cultural impact in Britain was clear, although the political impact was more muted. The impact of temperance varied by country with a clear north/south divide within Europe. In some countries, temperance was allied with medical professionals' concern about drink, and it is to the role of different professional interests and their impact on substances which we now turn.

4

The Professionals: Doctors and Pharmacists

Pharmacists were the key professional group controlling access to opiates. Their oral history reminiscences make this clear. Here are some who worked in the 1920s and 1930s speaking about how they dispensed opium.

'People came in regularly for paregoric (camphorated opium tincture), and chlorodyne, both Collis Browne's and Teasdale's. We sold all of them over the counter.'

'Mist Expect. And cough mixtures. We sold a lot of paregoric and opiate squills in those days. We could sell it over the counter.'

'A cough mixture...contained aniseed, peppermint, paregoric, laudaunum, a stick of black liquorice and a pound of black treacle. She (the maker) called it "All Fours".'

'We sold a lot of a preparation which was known as Infants Thunder. It was a bottle of nearly black stuff, with some laudanum in it, to put the kids to sleep.'[67]

Informal doctoring also provided access. Mrs Copper who lived in North Kensington in London used to run errands for her father, who provided doctoring of an unqualified sort for the local poor area.

She remembered,

my father you know, he worked for a licensed vet, a very clever man. And when my dad was a boy he worked for him...but he learned a lot. And he learned all about these medicines...You'd have to get a wine glass, you'd put so much, he'd know how much to give, so much water and it used to cure people in no time and they all used to come to him...He used to send me, I know, he'd give you ninepence, and I'd have to go to the chemist in Golborne Road, North Kensington, and buy three penn'orth of laudanum, three penn'orth of red lavender and three penn'orth essence of peppermint. Well that was for dysentery, diarrhoea and all that. The neighbours used to come to him for that.[68]

This chapter looks at the role of professional occupations such as pharmacy and medicine in imposing particular types of controls on, and 'ways of seeing' the different substances. In the last chapter, we looked at how a social movement, in that case temperance, could operate to help change culture and regulation. Temperance as a movement helped to develop new ways of thinking about drinking and also arguments about the role of the state. The nineteenth century also saw the 'rise of professional society', the increasing importance of middle-class professional occupations like medicine, with greater authority within society. Those professionals increasingly looked to the state as a means of establishing their own professional credentials. They also wanted the state to provide the means whereby professionals could treat and manage the conditions or practices which had been identified as appropriate for their intervention. Here we will look at how professionals became involved with opium and alcohol and the impact this had on deciding the paths these substances took within society—by contrast with tobacco, where there was, at this stage, relatively little professional involvement.

As opium moved away from completely open sale, and the popular culture of consumption which we looked at in the previous chapter, it came initially to form part of a system of pharmaceutical regulation. Pharmacists, not doctors, were initially the lead professionals in managing access to the drug and this system of pharmaceutical regulation lasted really until the First World War. A separate profession called pharmacy was in the process of organization in the UK and elsewhere in the mid nineteenth century, taking on board the existing chemists and druggists and the apothecaries, whose main concern was dispensing drugs. In the UK the professional body was the Pharmaceutical Society, which was set up in 1841. It thereafter sought government backing for its unique educational qualifications and for restriction of trade in the interests of its pharmacist members. Pharmacy Acts were passed in 1852 and in 1868 which set pharmacy on the road to this professional status. These Acts also began a process of controlling the sale of drugs. The 1851 Arsenic Act had already controlled sale of that drug, and the 1868 Act took things further. It put fifteen selected poisons into a two-part schedule. Drugs like cyanide of potassium and ergot (much used as an abortifacient) were in the first part of the schedule and were quite restricted. They could be sold only if the purchaser was known to the pharmacist or to an intermediate person who was known to both of them. There had to be a detailed entry in the poisons register and the container had to be clearly labelled 'poison', with the name of the product and the name and address of the seller on it. Drugs in the second part of the schedule had less restriction and only had to be labelled.

Opium was placed in this less restrictive second part of the schedule; the struggle over where it was to be placed and how regulated gives an indication of its important role in popular culture at the time. Pharmacists wanted the right to control the sale of such a popular and lucrative item—but they did not want restriction to be at such a level that their sales would be affected—or would perhaps continue in an unregulated way. It was the classic debate about the relationship between regulation and the creation of a potential black market. In this case, the danger was that dealers outside pharmacy might continue to take part of the trade. Throughout the 1850s and 1860s, there were debates about various bills brought forward to control the sale of poisons which illustrated this dilemma. There was a division of opinion between public health interests, which almost uniformly called for greater restriction, and pharmacists, who saw the realities of their own position. Pharmacists also realized that opium played a great role in the lives of the poor and even public health interests had to acknowledge this. Professor Arnold Taylor, leading pharmacologist, recognized the importance of small sales to working people. The way round, in his view, was a system—rather akin in some respects to the Gothenburg System we discussed in the previous chapter—whereby pennyworths to adults could still be sold without restriction but had to be drunk in the shop.[69] The Home Secretary of the day, Spencer Walpole, introducing one version of control in 1859, argued 'If you put difficulty in the way of giving it in small quantities to persons who desire it, you may interfere inconveniently with these requirements as well as with the trade of the chemist.'[70]

The draft version of what later became the 1868 Act at one stage dropped opium altogether from its coverage. Why was this? It was later revealed that this was because of protests from within the pharmaceutical profession itself. Elias Bremridge, its secretary, explained, 'the promoters of the Bill received such strong representations from chemists residing principally in Cambridgeshire, Lincolnshire and Norfolk, against interfering with their business—opium, as they stated, being one of their chief articles of trade'.[71] But in the end opium did appear, with labelling-only restrictions in the schedule to the Act; patent medicines were, however, excluded from control. There were other exclusions too. 'Preparations of opium' were controlled, 'preparations containing opium' were not. The former contained more than 1 per cent opium, but it meant that weaker popular preparations like paregoric could still be sold without restriction. Direct over-the-counter sales to members of the public continued, with the pharmacist rather than a general dealer in charge. Such was the interest in this regulation that in 2012 the novelist Anne Perry used the machinations round the 1868 Pharmacy Act as the plot line for one of her Victorian thrillers.[72]

Further controls over patent medicines were put in place in the 1890s. The main concern was about the product called chlorodyne (an amalgamation of the words 'chloroform' and 'anodyne'). There were many commercial cholorodynes on the market but the best-known product was Dr J. Collis Browne's version. Collis Browne had been a doctor working in India, where he first used the preparation. In 1848, while on leave, he went to the colliery village of Trimdon in County Durham to help fight an outbreak of cholera. Chlorodyne, his preparation, produced encouraging results. In 1856, when he left the army, he went into partnership with J. T. Davenport, a chemist in Great Russell Street in London, who gained the sole right to manufacture and market the compound. The product claimed to deal with an impressive range of ailments—'coughs, colds, influenza, diarrhoea, stomach chills, cholera, flatulence, bronchitis, croup, whooping cough, neuralgia and rheumatism'. The main ingredients were chloroform and morphine. Although it was sold as a patent medicine, Collis Browne had not in fact patented his product and so there were many attempts to find out the recipe and to market rival products. There were Towle's, Squire's, and Freeman's chlorodynes also on the market.

Patent medicines like these were popular at a time when many consumers still had little regular access to medicines through their doctors. The Revd W. R. Dawes, a country parson in Buckinghamshire, who gave free treatment to patients, wrote to Davenport in 1858 asking for fresh supplies.

> The trying weather lately having caused a large demand for this medicine, my stock is suddenly exhausted and I shall be particularly obliged by your sending me a *pint and half* of the Chlorodyne safely packed in a box by the *Oxford coach.*[73]

Sarah Williams of Portsmouth died in 1889 and was reported to have bought at least three bottles a week from her local branch of the Timothy Whites chemists chain. Here was an instance of a poor consumer who took too much. These cases multiplied in the professional journals in the 1880s and 1890s, and in 1892 a successful Treasury prosecution of Davenport's meant that chlorodyne had to come under the provisions of the 1868 Pharmacy Act. Henceforth, it was to be labelled 'poison' and sold by pharmacists rather than by general dealers.

So by the end of the nineteenth century, opium and allied patent medicines came under a system of pharmaceutical regulation. This was a system which formalized access and sale, but did not aim to do anything further. Its roots lay in professional self-organization, but also in alliances between pharmacy, medical and public health interests who were concerned to do something about the problems of over-the-counter sale and consequent levels of accidental overdosing. In this system, opium was recognized as a self-help product, one with both medical and social uses, but it was essentially an item of consumption which needed relatively limited professional controls. In other countries in Europe, control by pharmacists also seems to have been the norm in the nineteenth century, and there is evidence of this in Germany, France, and the Netherlands, although the role of the doctor's prescription as a means of controlling access seems to have become important at an earlier date—in the 1870s in Germany for example.[74] Studies of the role of pharmacy as a route for access in the USA also imply that a doctor's prescription was necessary.[75] This seems to have been less the case in the UK at least until the time of further controls during and after the First World War. The widespread evidence of popular 'over the counter' use may mark the UK out from other European countries, or it may simply be that oral evidence was never gathered there while consumers were still alive.

Meanwhile a rather different system of control was emergent from a different professional grouping. This was the medical profession, which, like pharmacy, was establishing its professional standing in the nineteenth century, in its case in the UK through the 1858 Medical Act and the formation of the General Medical Council. Ideas about disease solidified in the second half of the century, in particular after the advent of germ theory, and it became possible to identify and categorize particular types of disease. One disease view which came to the fore was the view that compulsive alcohol and drug use was itself a form of 'disease'. In the early 1880s the first professional British medical society aimed at promoting this idea and the role of professionals concerned with it came into being.

On 25 February 1884, a meeting was held at 1 Adam Street, in the Adelphi in London. Chaired by Dr Norman Kerr, prominent both as a temperance reformer and also as the Medical Officer of Health for Marylebone since 1874, the meeting resolved to form an association with the title of the 'Society for the Study and Cure of Inebriety'. The objects of the new society were loosely defined as being 'to investigate the various causes of inebriety, and to educate the professional and public mind to a recognition of the physical aspects of habitual intemperance'. Two months later, on 25 April 1884, a luncheon at the rooms of the Medical Society of London formally inaugurated the newly established Society. The company was prestigious, including Lord Shaftesbury, the Bishop of Ripon, and nearly a hundred doctors, including the presidents of four medical societies. After lunch Norman Kerr delivered a presidential address which focused on some of the key themes which lay behind the Society's formation and which were to guide its work until the end of the century. 'Inebriety' was first and foremost a disease.

> Inebriety is for the most part the issue of certain physical conditions, is an offspring of material parentage, is the natural product of a depraved, debilitated, or defective nervous organization. Whatever else it may be, in a host of cases it is a true disease, as unmistakeably a disease as is gout or epilepsy or insanity.[76]

The disease concept was advanced as an alternative to criminalization of the drinker, to the penal approach. Treatment in a hospital or inebriate asylum was to be actively promoted in opposition to confinement in prison.

> We shall be satisfied if we succeed in impressing on the public mind that inebriates are not necessarily scoundrels—that to treat the dipsomaniac as a criminal is not to cure but to confirm his inebriety, not to reform him but to make him worse—that no reproach should be cast on the inebriate for surrendering his freedom in the hope of cure-that no slur should be attached to residence (voluntary or involuntary) in a Home for Inebriates any more than in a hospital or asylum.

Kerr was of the opinion that the state had a role in establishing a system of treatment in institutions and ensuring the pauper and working-class drinkers were able to gain access as well as those who were better off.

> [I]t is the duty of the State to make permanent, while amending, the present temporary Act for promoting the reformation and cure of

the habitual drunkard, and to supply adequate provision for the care and treatment of such needy disease inebriates as, from their serious illness of body and mind, are unable to contribute to their own maintenance and support.

These three ideas dominated the Society's early work: advocacy of a disease view of inebriety as the scientific alternative to what was seen as an outmoded moralistic approach; medical concepts and approaches as an humane alternative to imprisonment; and the belief that the state and the medical profession should work together to achieve these ends. Inebriety was the dominant concept in the UK and the USA at the end of the nineteenth century, bringing together alcohol and drugs.

The Society's original optimism was shown in its title although the 'cure' had been dropped by the end of the 1880s. It had its origins in another organization, the Society for Promoting Legislation for the Control and Cure of Habitual Drunkards, which had been formed in 1876 by a group of doctors and a lawyer, and of which Kerr was also president. The Society's belief was that treatment and also some form of state-funded treatment system was needed to enable drunkards and, to a lesser extent, drug takers, to be taken out of the ambit of the law courts where they often ended up. This was an objective which united the interest group around inebriety and there were high hopes that it could be achieved.

On 19 September 1885, a special train ran from Euston station in London to Rickmansworth, then a country town. It carried a mixed party of doctors, clergymen, temperance abstainers, and prohibitionists, many of whom were members of the Society for the Study of Inebriety. They were attending a reception at the Dalrymple Home, a licensed inebriates retreat run by the Homes for Inebriates Association. The guest of honour was Dr Joseph Parrish, president of the American Association for the Study and Cure of Inebriety, founded in 1870, before the British Society. A resolution was passed that day congratulating Parrish and his group 'on the steadily increasing recognition of the diseased condition of the confirmed drunkard, and on the generous provision for the treatment of the poorest of this class in America at the public expense'.

The day's enthusiastic outing resulted in part from the concern about alcohol rather than drugs, but the two substances were becoming yoked together through this agitation and the plans for reform. Public concern as we saw in the last chapter was expressed through the temperance movement, which had become by the late nineteenth century a substantial working-class movement in many countries, English speaking and Nordic ones above all. But public concern also took other forms, notably in the movement to provide medical state-funded treatment for inebriates. Its intention was to divert 'habitual drunkards' out of the 'revolving door' of prison and into treatment; its rationale was that drinkers were diseased. Modern scientific research had revealed 'that intemperance has a physical and pathological as well as a legal, moral and spiritual aspect, that there is a gospel of the body as there is a gospel of the soul', stated Norman Kerr, in an 1893 lecture on inebriety and jurisprudence.[77]

In Britain, the classic punishment for drunkenness at the time was a fine, or imprisonment for several weeks or months. The number of those imprisoned had risen rapidly, from 4,000 in the early 1860s to 23,000 in 1876. There were moves to reform this process and to insert medicine into it. In 1870, Donald Dalrymple, Liberal Member of Parliament for Bath, formerly a surgeon in Norwich and proprietor of the Heigham Lunatic Asylum, unsuccessfully introduced a private member's bill. Two years later, a parliamentary select committee on the control and management of habitual drunkards, of which Dalrymple was chairman, urged legislation to bring about the compulsory treatment of voluntary patients and of convicted drunkards. The results were initially disappointing. In 1879, the Habitual Drunkards Act made treatment of non-criminal inebriates available only to those who could pay. A further act followed in 1888. The Inebriates Act of 1898 allowed the committal of criminal inebriates to state-funded reformatories if they were tried and convicted of drunkenness four times in one year. But what medical reformers wanted, the compulsory power to detain non-criminal inebriates, never became law. Even the small amount of change which was achieved in law translated only with difficulty into actual provision on the ground. Financial battles between the Home Office and the local authorities, charged with funding the reformatories, blighted the implementation of the Act.

But the Acts brought drinking and drug taking together (although not smoking).[78] The provisions of the Acts covered drug taking as well as alcohol, as long as the substance was ingested by drinking it. Inebriety was classified according to the intoxicating agent: 'we thus have alcohol, opium, chloral, ether, chlorodyne, and other forms of the disease'. Laudanum tippling was covered, but not drugs that were injected. A later (1908) departmental committee on the inebriates acts accepted that all drug taking should be included. It also proposed that an inebriate, thus defined, could apply to have an appointed guardian, a strategy derived from lunacy legislation, whereby the guardian would decide where the inebriate would live, deprive him of intoxicants, and warn sellers of drink and drugs against supplying him. After a warning had been given, any supply to a drinker or drug taker would be an offence. Provision for compulsion was in place if voluntary control proved insufficient.

Plans to extend the law in this way were by then a faint hope. Even before the First World War, inebriates legislation fell into disuse. Only fourteen reformatories, dealing with 4,590 inmates, were then still in operation. Drinkers and drug takers were covered by legislation dealing with lunacy and mental deficiency.

The power to commit offenders to inebriate reformatories was heavily implemented in cases of neglect and child cruelty. The 1902 Licensing Act enabled a magistrate to send an inebriate wife to a reformatory in place of a separation order. The Provision of Meals Act of 1903 and Prevention of Cruelty Act of 1904 provided for detention when neglect and cruelty were due to drink and were also used to commit drunken prostitutes and the poorest and most troublesome section of the male labouring classes. Such sections of society, according to Branthwaite, the inspector of reformatories,

> bring into the world ill-fed, uncared-for, and mentally useless children, who provide the mass from which the future criminal, drunken, and lunatic army is recruited.

At the turn of the nineteenth century, reformers were concerned with 'the future of the race', the transmission of the disease of alcoholism from one generation to another, and the hereditary taint, the 'alcohol gene' of its day, of alcoholism. Women were disproportionately represented among those who were confined and we will return to look at their role in the next chapter on 'fear'.

The mandate of the institutions encompassed reform, rehabilitation, and punishment. Offenders were kept away from the temptations of the city (hence Rickmansworth, which was then a country town, for the Dalrymple Retreat) and confined for a lengthy period—between one and three years—as compared with one to three months in prison. Cure involved physical, mental, and moral rehabilitation. Dr F. J. Gray of Old Park Hall Retreat in Staffordshire described his methods in 1888:

> In the cricket season we have a half-day's match every week…often some medical men and clergymen come up for tennis, so that there are plenty of means both for exercise and amusement on the premises…we begin the day with prayers…and finish the day with prayers. Breakfast at nine o'clock, which consists of porridge (to which I attach a great importance), bacon and dried fish, varied with eggs, sausages, bread, butter, jam, and marmalade.

Enthusiasm for such treatment was international and the 'inebriety model' was widely accepted in professional groupings in the UK and USA. In America, the temperance-based Washingtonian movement of the first half of the nineteenth century had founded small, private institutions dedicated to the moral treatment of voluntary patients. Promoters of the asylum model, some organized through the American Association for the Cure of Inebriety, wanted institutions that were large, public, rural, and capable of holding and disciplining the inmates. The concept of the 'industrial hospital' argued for in the 1890s failed because jails were seen to have the same function for less cost. Public institutions specifically for drinkers did not gain ground in the USA. The Massachusetts State Hospital for Dipsomaniacs and Inebriates was plagued by patient escapes, rebellions, and the accumulation of chronic cases. The advent of prohibition in the 1920s seemed to substitute prevention for cure.

In English-speaking countries and in Germany, the popularity of inebriate institutions peaked in the years before 1914. In the Nordic countries, the peak of interest was later, from 1910 to 1935. There were inebriate asylums in Australia and South Africa. After the First World War, with restrictions on opening hours and reduction of the strength of alcohol, prosecutions fell in England. The alcohol problem was no longer the central question, and inebriate reformatories seemed less relevant. Different trends had emerged in psychiatry. The prestige of mental-asylum doctors was eroded, and a middle-class clientele was sought outside the asylum. The legacy in English-speaking countries was apparently minimal. Systems for handling alcoholism continued in Sweden and Switzerland, although these were less medically oriented. Both countries arrived in the period between the wars at a three-tiered system of community agencies, hospitals, and work camps. Physicians relinquished compulsory handling of cases, seeing these cases as 'social' rather than 'medical'.

In practical terms, the emergent alliance between medical experts and the state over inebriety had achieved little by the outbreak of the war. But the theories which had been developed since the eighteenth century about the overuse of alcohol (drugs to a lesser extent) as a disease were of great importance and continued in medical and popular currency. In effect, with variations and modifications, they have continued to underpin dominant medical views about drink and, to a lesser extent, drugs, into the present day. They have also modified public views about 'drugs' as well. People involved in the addictions field like to look back to antecedents and it used to be argued that a modern concept of 'addiction' developed or was 'discovered' in America towards the end of the eighteenth century.[79] The American physician Benjamin Rush published his *Inquiry in the Effects of Ardent Spirits on the Human Body and Mind* in 1784. Thomas Trotter was an English counterpart, often also hailed as the originator of disease views of alcoholism. He published *An Essay Medical, Philosophical and Chemical on Drunkenness and its Effects on the Human Body,* in 1804. Trotter saw the habit of drunkenness as a 'disease of the mind' with a particular role for the medical profession.

More recently this view of 'firsts' has been challenged and several historians have pointed out that such discussions about disease and alcohol were also common in the eighteenth century among many other writers. In fact the key features of the concept had been developed throughout that century and were more or less in place by the 1770s. They were part of ongoing debates about the relationship between the body and the mind and about the moral implications of the relationship. Drink provided an admirable case study for these discussions.[80] Before Trotter, John Coakley Lettsom had already presented a detailed study of the physical effects of drink. Lettsom described the cycle, leading from tippling for stimulus, relief, or exhilaration; to low-spirits, which were the inevitable after-effects; which in turn could be obliterated only by further bouts of yet heavier drinking. He cited as an example

> those of delicate habits, who have endeavoured to overcome their nervous debility by the aid of spirits: many of these have begun the use of these poisons from persuasion of their utility, rather than from love of them: the relief, however, being temporary, to keep up their effects, frequent access is had to the same delusion, till at length what was taken by compulsion, gains attachment, and a little drop of brandy, or gin and water, becomes as necessary as food; the female sex, from natural delicacy, acquire this custom by small degrees, and the poison being admitted in small doses, is slow in its operations, but not less painful in its effects.[81]

Both Lettsom and Rush developed what they called a 'moral and physical thermometer' which put consuming small beer, cider, perry, wine, porter, and even strong beer in 'moderate quantities' on the right side of temperance, drawing the line at punch, toddy, grog, rum, and whisky.

What was different about the late eighteenth-century and early nineteenth-century declarations of Rush and Trotter, so the historian Roy Porter has persuasively argued, was not the theories themselves, but the fertile context in which theories found themselves. Evangelical Christianity, the moral movement of temperance, the expanding ambitions of the state, all provided fertile ground for ideas of disease to take root.

One can track a path forward from these declarations. During the first half of the nineteenth century European theoreticians elaborated the disease concept in various ways. The connection with expanding theories about insanity was a strong one. In 1819 the German von Bruhl Cramer argued that habitual drunkenness was a disease of the nervous system, a pre-existing condition, which produced the craving for alcohol which he called 'dipsomania'. The French alienist (or mental illness specialist) Esquirol contended in the 1830s that there was a mental disease which manifested itself in the inability to abstain from intoxicating liquors. He classified it as a form of monomania, a category he had invented where the patient was unable to reason on one particular subject but was otherwise lucid. At the middle of the nineteenth century, the Swedish Magnus Huss provided clinical descriptions of a condition he labelled 'chronic alcoholism'.[82] By the 1850s many British doctors had begun to accept some form of disease theory, among them Alexander Peddie, who was an enthusiastic proponent of the new theory. Early physiological enquiry into alcohol by investigators such as W. B. Carpenter, lecturer in physiology at the London Hospital, began to link research into the effects of alcohol with theories about habituation. Carpenter reported on trials of hard work where drink was either consumed or not—among farm workers and also among brickmakers, with productivity higher among the teetotallers.[83]

Carpenter, like Kerr later on in the Society for the Study of Inebriety, mixed moral and medical imperatives.

> [W]hilst there are adequate medical reasons for Abstinence from the *habitual* use of even a 'moderate' quantity of Alcoholic liquor, there are also strong moral grounds for Abstinence, from that occasional use of them, which is too frequently thought to be requisite for social enjoyment.[84]

This mixing of moral and medical also derived from concepts within insanity, for example Prichard's concept of 'moral insanity' and carried over to discussion of inebriety. Kerr's own inaugural address to the Society was unclear as to whether he was talking about vice, sin, crime, or disease.

The rise of these medicalized models of drunkenness and inebriety has been interpreted by some historians, influenced by the ideas of the French philosopher Michel Foucault, as examples of the extension of the 'clinical gaze' and the control of populations through making deviant activities medical and pathological. But there was no unified theory of drunkenness as disease and in part this was because 'inebriety' did not fit well within ideas about rationality and reason. Inebriates were both rational and insane.[85]

Inebriety was also closely allied, at least at its outset, with temperance views and many of the early medical members of the Society were also temperance supporters. Some also moved easily between temperance and anti-opium agitations. Benjamin Ward Richardson was a member of the SSI and also a temperance lecturer and active in the National Temperance League.[86] The toast at the first meeting of the SSI was to 'the temperance organizations'. The disease view was part of the moves among the medical profession in these years to drop the medical use of alcohol. Ideas about disease were linked also to the late Victorian focus on 'degeneration of the race' which we will examine in the next chapter on 'fear'.

Inebriety was important as an idea because it linked drink and drugs together—although not tobacco, which when discussed, was seen as a 'habit' rather than as a disease. Tobacco did not fall within any of the legal systems which had led to the inebriety model for alcohol and drugs, and social attitudes towards it were also more tolerant. No one was being sent to prison for excessive tobacco use as they were for alcohol consumption. Liquid opiates were covered by the terms of the existing Acts and from the 1880s the Society was also pushing to include injected opiates, primarily morphine, as well. Bringing all opiate-based drugs in all forms within the concept of 'inebriety' would have important consequences for yoking the two substances together.

But there was also a different strand of theorizing about drugs also coming into play from the 1870s; and its dissemination helps to explain the subsequent divergence in thinking about alcohol and drugs and disease. Ideas came from European writers initially and were specifically focused on the hypodermic injection of morphia and its effects. We will be discussing the advent of the opium alkaloids and technical developments such as the syringe in Chapter 6. These technical developments led to a distinctive way of writing about the effects of drugs which did not fit within 'inebriety'. Dr Edward Levinstein of Berlin was the first European writer whose work reached the British medical profession. He published *Die Morphiumsucht nacht Eigenen Beobachtungen* in German in 1877 and it was translated the following year as *Morbid Craving for Morphia*. The book was based on his own experiences in the institutional treatment of morphine addiction in Berlin and was important in defining what he called 'morphinism' as a separate condition or disease. 'Morphinismus', 'morphia delirium' and 'morphia evil' had been in use as terms. Levinstein claimed to be the first to define the condition as a disease similar to dipsomania, although not fully a mental illness. He still saw it as a human passion, 'such as smoking, gambling, greediness for profit, sexual excesses, etc'. Another German physician, Dr H. Obersteiner, published articles on 'chronic morphinism' in the journal (newly established) *Brain* in the late 1870s. Dr Albrecht Erlenmeyer's work on morphine addiction was published in German in 1879 but became known in English towards the end of the 1880s.

To these European writers was added an Anglo-American strand by the last decades of the century. They sometimes talked about 'morphia habit' and sometimes about morphinomania, a condition akin to insanity. Dr Seymour Sharkey, a British doctor, wrote about a patient of his, a manager in the city, who had used the drug over a seventeen-year period. He later expanded his views in an article in the magazine *Nineteenth Century* in 1887. Oscar Jenning's work on what he called the 'morphia habit' was voluminous towards the end of the century. An ex-morphine addict himself, English by background, the bulk of his case histories came from France. In the early years of the twentieth-century, American influence was significant. T. D. Crothers' *Morphinism and Narcomanias from other Drugs* was published in 1902 and J. B. Mattison's *The Mattison Method in Morphinism: A Modern and Humane Treatment of the Morphin Disease* (1902) crossed the Atlantic. Mattison spoke and wrote for the Society for the Study of Inebriety. This language of emergent 'addiction' tended to separate drugs and alcohol.

Not all medical writers used this language. The leading British physician T. C. Allbutt's text book *Systems of Medicine*, which went through many editions, used the terminology of 'opium poisoning' to which was added the words 'and other intoxications'. This framing was still in use in 1906, when Allbutt had been joined as editor by the pharmacologist W. E. Dixon, later to play a key role in the formation of a separate British drug policy. The texts which still used ideas about 'poisoning' would divide their discussion into two sections—'acute poisoning' which was the overdose, accidental or otherwise, and what they called 'chronic poisoning', which was the 'habit' in other phraseology. This divergence was important because it linked medical ideas to those also common in pharmaceutical regulation. The language was much more neutral in tone than the moral/medical formulations which marked both inebriety and the emergent morphine discourse. It talked about managing a condition rather than treating a disease.

Increasingly, however, the language of a separate condition called 'addiction' was applied to drugs as a whole, certainly by the outbreak of the First World War. Medical writers talked about 'morphinomanias and inebriety' well into the 1900s, while Norman Kerr's standard text *Inebriety, its Etiology, Pathology, Treatment and Jurisprudence* first published under that title in the late 1880s, was republished as *Inebriety: or Narcomania* in 1894. What was happening during the 1890s and early 1900s, slowly but surely, was the decline of inebriety and the emergence of a separate set of ideas about morphinomania or narcomania, applied to all opiate substances—but not to drink. An analysis of the terminology used in leading medical journals, the *Lancet* and the *British Medical Journal* in the late nineteenth and early decades of the twentieth century, shows that the term alcoholism came into use, but that it, along with the term 'inebriety', was in decline by the time of the First World War.[87] By 1914, the language of 'addiction' was taking precedence. Sir Ronald Armstrong Jones, for example, a distinguished mental health specialist, wrote of 'Drug addiction in relation to mental disorder' in the *British Journal of Inebriety* in 1914. This was not just semantic nicety but indicated a new modernism, what the historian Tim Hickman has called a cultural crisis of modernity which ideas about addiction helped both to support and to create. There were also legal reasons for the divergence. Morphine injection could not be part of the inebriates legislation because the mode of ingestion was not through drinking. Although there was medical pressure for this formulation to be changed, the argument about including injectable morphine was not accepted until 1908—by which time inebriety as a means of managing alcohol and drug users, was going out of fashion both intellectually and in practical ways. Addiction was emergent as a 'drugs only' concept reinforced by technology and, as we will see in Chapter 7, by later international developments as well.

However, we should not assume that these models necessarily applied in all countries. Inebriety was an Anglo-American concept but it was little, if at all, discussed in other European countries. In Scandinavia a social model prevailed and doctors were much less involved. In Italy, the terminology was not used, nor was 'addiction' in use. In that country the impetus for disease views came from forensic scientists rather than public health doctors or mental health specialists.[88] Which professional group claimed authority also helped define the nature of the concepts.

Along with disease of all sorts went treatment. Early writers on 'addiction' who saw it as more or less a bad habit had seen nothing wrong in withdrawing the substance abruptly and without substitution. Professor Christison, for example, the Edinburgh pharmacologist who believed that opium eating and longevity could go together, saw nothing wrong in withdrawing the drug suddenly. Levinstein later on also favoured abrupt withdrawal. The addict was to be treated in a locked and barred room and guarded night and day by male warder nurses. But the biggest area of debate—and professional self-affirmation—was over gradual withdrawal, or substitution treatment. This was a common area of discussion in the alcohol field. Drugs used to detoxify and treat alcoholic inebriates from the 1860s into the 1930s included other agents such as whisky and beer; *Cannabis indica*; chloral hydrate; paraldehyde; veronal and other sedatives; coca; hyoscyamus; belladonna; and atropine.[89] For drugs, too, rapid, semi-rapid and gradual methods were popular.

Because of the 'poisoning' model in the medical text books, the ways of dealing with addiction were sometimes close to the treatment of an opium overdose. For example, atropine was also a way of dealing with opium poisoning. Norman Kerr had originally used abrupt methods but later converted to using potassium and sodium bromide over a period of a month to subdue irritability. Some doctors used cannabis, others coca. Methods rose and declined dependent on what was in favour. Cocaine was much lauded in the 1880s but the subject of dire medical warnings by the 1900s. Physical antidotes were also recommended—the removal of decayed teeth which were supposed to poison the whole system, was often recommended.

There were also commercial cures on the market, which paralleled those patent medicines based on opium. The 'Normyl' cure for Alcohol and Drug Addictions (24 days medicine in 24 bottles) was composed of 75 per cent alcohol with strychnine. The Teetolia treatment (after years of drink and drug taking—cured in four days) had alcohol and quinine. There was the Keeley Cure, and the St George association for the Cure of the Morphia Habit. The Turvey treatment for alcoholism and narcomania was 'earning the gratitude of the nation, the support of the Ministry, the thankfulness of hundreds of our most successful business and literary men of the day'.[90] The Malayan anti-opium plant, *Combretum sundaicum*, also attracted much interest in the medical journals in the 1900s.

Alcohol and drugs were firmly set within this 'disease and treatment' model by the end of the nineteenth century. But in recent times, they have both been termed 'public health' issues, and of course, smoking has been a recent public health concern par excellence. So did the substances fit within a public health model in the nineteenth century? The answer is only to a limited extent. Drink, drugs, and tobacco were not major public health issues, and, in the case of tobacco, not a public health issue at all. The public health movement in the nineteenth century focused on sanitation and on cleansing the environment. Public health was driven by theories of miasma, the atmospheric transmission of disease, rather than, as later, by germ theory, and so the role of drink and drugs was rather muted. Drink was a matter of concern, but as Brian Harrison noted, the all-encompassing nature of the temperance movement as the vehicle for anti-drink agitation, meant that drink was not really a public health issue. Opium use was mentioned in public health reports, not least Edwin Chadwick's famous *On the Sanitary Condition of the Labouring Population* (1842). It also figured largely in the reports made by Sir John Simon as Medical Officer to the Privy Council in the 1860s. Reports on infant mortality especially in the Fens, carried out by his medical investigators, were among the first consistent medical investigations into adult as well as infant mortality from opiates. The publication of the Registrar General's mortality reports also raised the issue of deaths from opium, usually accidental. So drink and drugs were of tangential interest to public health and some of the early supporters of the SSI (including Kerr, who was a Medical Officer of Health) were public health professionals. The treatment aim of segregating the diseased drunkard or opium taker in an institution had parallels with the public health strategy of notification and isolation, which came into being in the 1880s to isolate sufferers from epidemic disease. But there was no discussion at this point about drug use being 'infectious' as there would be later on, in the 1960s. So the model of public health had little application to the substances at this point. They travelled down a road of medicalization, but the relationship with public health was slight.

The role of professionalization for drink and drugs thus brought two professions—pharmacy and the emergent specialities of mental health—to the fore. By the beginning of the twentieth-century drugs were beginning to go down the route of the 'addiction' concept which to some extent brought a divergence with drink.

But the role of professional control was different for both alcohol and tobacco. Both retained a substantial non-professional area of availability and consequent different styles of regulation. Pharmacy had a role to play for both these substances. Pharmacists sold both tobacco and alcohol as the advertisements in pharmacists' shop windows reveal.

Oral histories taken from pharmacists show that tobacco was often in the form of snuff. One who worked in an industrial area in the 1930s recalled:

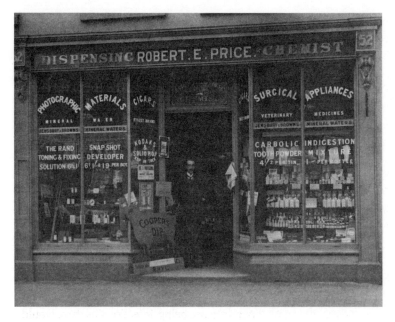

FIGURE 4 Chemist's shop with advertisements for tobacco in the window.

The mill-workers would call in on their way to or from work—or occasionally at lunchtime—and buy 3d [3 pence] worth of snuff [1/4 oz]. Often they didn't bother to ask for it. They would just hold up three fingers, or else come up to the counter and sniff. Some of them wanted it mixed with menthol. We would charge a penny extra for it. Tiny crystals of menthol would be ground up with the snuff.

Preparing the snuff was the job of the apprentice in the 1930s. Alan Kendall, the pharmacist, continues:

We weighed out a lot of snuff, which was powdered tobacco. We got through 14 pounds [7 kilograms] at a time. It arrived packed in one pound tins. It was weighed out into quarter ounce and half ounce quantities. We wrapped it in pages from the *Chemist and Druggist*, which were cut into quarters. We made cornet-shaped holders. We put the snuff into it and folded down the top.

With the introduction of the National Health Service in the UK in 1948 the number of pharmacies holding tobacco licences diminished as the dispensing of prescriptions became a much more lucrative activity, but trade in tobacco products continued. Indeed, in some parts of the country chemists' shops with integral off-licences and tobacconists were seen as natural partners.[91]

But both substances also retained a substantial area of lay availability, albeit regulated. The publican fulfilled an extensive social role, with licensed drinking places for all types of customer. Pubs provided meeting places and centres for recreation; public lavatories were provided, lodgings for homeless or itinerant men and a place to stay for lodgers who were only allowed in their lodgings to sleep. Harrison's words sum it up:

> The drink shop's blaze of light and lavish baroque facade were thrown into relief by the meanness of its immediate surroundings: by poor street lighting and dark homes where candles could not be afforded. Yet the drinkseller was no parasitic villain: he responded to a genuine human need, and was a popular and respected provider of recreation and comfort to a world which would have been intolerably drab without him.[92]

Pharmacy had a role for drink but this was as nothing compared to the role of the publican. For tobacco the role of the retail tobacconist was also important as a means of lay control of access. There were half a million licensed dealers by the 1930s in the UK and by that date, they had one of the strongest retail trade associations. The nineteenth-century tobacconist developed in two ways from earlier craft skills. Some continued to sell a range of tobacco while others only sold pre-packaged products through general stores and kiosks.[93]

So, for both those substances, lay licensed control and access remained of major importance. Opiates by contrast, had already by the end of the nineteenth century gone down a much more professionalized route. The pharmacist was still centre stage before the First World War, although doctors with their prescription pads and ideas about disease and treatment systems were an increasingly important force. But the question of who consumed substances as well as who provided them commercially or professionally, was also an important underlying issue and this concern, allied with fear, is the subject of the next chapter.

5
Fear: Dens and Degeneration

He is in the meanest and closest of small rooms. Through the ragged window curtain, the light of early day steals in from a miserable court. He lies, dressed, across a large unseemly bed, upon a bedstead that has indeed given way under the weight upon it. Lying, also dressed and also across the bed, not longwise, are a Chinaman, a Lascar, and a haggard woman. The two first are in a sleep or stupor; the last is blowing at a kind of pipe, to kindle it. And as she blows, and shading it with her lean hand, concentrates its red spark of light, it serves in the dim morning as a lamp to show him what he sees of her.

'Another?' says this woman, in a querulous, rattling whisper. 'Have another?'[94]

Charles Dickens' description of the opium den in his novel *The Mystery of Edwin Drood* was published in 1870. It followed a visit by the novelist himself and his American friend Fields to Bluegate Fields, an area of East London which other 'outsiders' had also visited and written about. Dickens' melodramatic presentation of opium smoking began a period when opium became associated with mystery and evil, with degrading and demoralizing effects on both English and Chinese smokers and in particular on the women who were involved.

This chapter uses the image of the opium den and the fears it evoked in the late nineteenth and early twentieth centuries to illustrate a further factor which should be evaluated in our consideration of the differential paths taken by the substances. That factor is fear. If substances evoke that emotion, through becoming connected, in the minds of the public or of the state, with feared or despised minorities, or appear to embody some threat, then regulation and cultural change may not be far behind. Once the substance is connected specifically with groups not mainstream in society, the discussion embodies a distancing and fear of 'the other'. Users and use are no longer in the mainstream but confined to deviant minorities. As many commentators on drugs have noted, who is using the substance is always an important issue in defining forms of response. A harsher response is more acceptable if the user is not like 'us'. The association of use with minorities both reflects but also reinforces, that process of marginalization—in culture and also in policy. This chapter will look at how racial minorities and also women began to fulfil the 'fear' role in the late nineteenth century, and at the different impact this had across the substances in the period just before the First World War. The association which began then has echoed down the years. In later chapters, we will see how similar fears have shaped responses to substances—including tobacco—in recent times.

The number of Chinese settling in London had begun to increase quite rapidly in the 1860s. In 1861, there were an estimated 147 Chinese in the whole country; by 1881 there were 665. Another influx came just prior to the First World War. Most lived in London, in the East End, in Stepney and Poplar. London's 'Chinatown' of the late nineteenth century was a small area by comparison with its American counterparts. The Chinese who settled in England serviced Chinese seamen by establishing laundries, shops, grocers, restaurants, and lodging houses. Their American counterparts were engaged in railroad construction, company mining, farming, or were employed in the nascent manufacturing industries of San Francisco. The centre of British settlement lay in two narrow dockland streets, Pennyfields and Limehouse Causeway. The Chinese were an isolated community.

Opium smoking as a practice had been talked about in English literary circles through the publication of 'travellers' tales' about the Far East, which wrote of it as an exotic, oriental practice. Only with the advent of greater numbers of Chinese in the country did descriptions of it as a domestic habit begin to surface. At first the tone was calm, but after Dickens' portrayal, the melodrama heightened. In the popular press, in social investigation, such as Blanchard Jerrold and Gustave Dore's London, A Pilgrimage (1872), in fictional and literary presentations, East End opium smoking underwent a change of image.[95] Powerful literary presentation helped, for example in Oscar Wilde's The Picture of Dorian Gray (1891) or in the Sherlock Holmes stories.[96]

> Through the gloom one could dimly catch a glimpse of bodies lying in strange fantastic poses, bowed shoulders, bent knees, heads thrown back and chins pointing upwards, with here and there a dark lack lustre eye turned upon the newcomer. Out of the black shadows there glimmered little red circles of light, now bright, now faint, as the burning poison waxed or waned in the bowls of the metal pipes. The most lay silent, but some muttered to themselves, and others talked together in a strange, low monotonous voice, their conversation coming in gushes, and then suddenly tailing off into silence, each mumbling out his own thoughts and paying little heed to the words of his neighbour.

This is from the Sherlock Holmes adventure, The Man with the Twisted Lip, also published in 1891.[97]

Such representations could be multiplied—they are part, even now, of our popular understanding of the vanished world of the mysterious East End at the turn of the century. But two questions can be asked: why did this imagery surface at the time it did—and what relationship did the brooding image bear to reality?

The imagery was part of a more general fashion for investigating the 'lower depths' of society in London from the 1870s which came to a peak in the 1890s and 1900s. In part this was related to the unease of respectable society at the potential 'threat' from working-class London revealed in the 1880s. The exposés of Andrew Mearns in his Bitter Cry of Outcast London (1883) or G. R. Sims in How the Poor Live showed how overcrowding and the housing crisis were bringing the poor and the criminal classes together. The existence of a 'residuum' of chronically poor and unemployed people was shown to be substantial and growing. Herded into slums, this threatening group was poised to engulf civilized

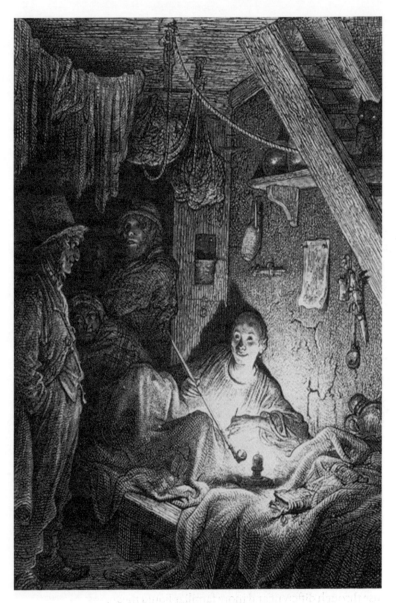

FIGURE 5 The popular image of the 'opium den'.

London.[98] The social investigations of Charles Booth in the same decade added fuel to this fever of fear about impending doom. Theories of urban degeneration coloured social debate about the condition of the urban poor. Social pollution was feared and a more general imagery of the fog that shrouded the East End of London symbolized the fears of respectable society; the fog of opium smoking was part of this fear.

Further fear came from two directions: the association of opium smoking with the organized movement against opium in the Far East—and its expanding connection with white men and women. For the anti-opiumists, opium smoking in China was categorized as a nonmedical form of use, whose results were always degrading and demoralizing and which led to inevitable addiction. These anti-opium arguments were also applied to the Chinese in the East End of London. East End Chinese, like those in China itself, should be 'saved' from their vice, so they argued. England's duty was also to the Chinese in England.

> Vile, uninhabitable tenements, transformed into the homes of vicious, ruinous indulgence…constitute a pitfall and a trap to many of those simple Easterns…Has England no duty here? Have those ill-paid servants no claim upon our care?[99]

Many of those arguing against opium smoking in the Far East made the journey to Limehouse to see the practice for themselves—and came away condemning it, as might have been expected. In fact a common view about the practice began to emerge and this was of importance for the detachment of opium from the 'normal' spectrum of use. There was agreement that moderate use was impossible, addiction inevitable, and moral and physical decline the invariable result.

> So powerful is its fascination, so fatal its hold, that loss of time, deferred expectancy, the trouble of preparation, nothing can win from the irresistible craving, which, once felt, so rarely loosens its grip.[100]

This view of opium smoking was different to the toleration of opiate use through different and more familiar liquid means.

Fear of the Chinese was also tied to wider concerns about immigration in the early twentieth century. This was a fear primarily directed at Jewish immigration into East London, but also took on board the Chinese and their alien 'practices'. Chinese seamen were often willing to work for lower rates of pay. In May 1908, there were bitter clashes in East India Dock Road when a picket led by the seamens' leader Havelock Wilson tried to ensure that Chinese sailors could not reach the Board of Trade offices and that only English crews were signed on. This led to an outpouring of complaints about Chinese practices in the local press of the time. In a comparison with Jewish immigrants the Chinese came off worst in the eyes of some commentators. An LCC inspector who had visited the Chinese area in 1904 pointed out that

> oriental cunning and cruelty...was hall-marked on every countenance...Until my visit to the Asiatic Sailors' Home, I had always considered some of the Jewish inhabitants of Whitechapel to be the worst type of humanity I had ever seen.

But the Chinese visit had beaten that. In the opium den itself, the 'loathsome apartment' where the drug was prepared led to smoking rooms where seamen lay 'dazed and helpless, jabbering in an incoherent manner'.[101]

The greatest fear about Chinese immigration and opium smoking was the connection with urban degeneration. The practice could spread more widely in society and pollute not just the working class, the fear with the general discussions about degeneration, but the middle-class population, undermining will and drive. Professor Goldwin Smith, speaking at an anti-opium meeting in Manchester in 1882, drew attention to Chinese immigration into America, Canada, and Australia as well as England bringing with them 'a hideous and very infectious vice'. The fear was that middle-class stock would degenerate through involvement with opium smoking; Oscar Wilde's *Dorian Gray* epitomized this fear. C. W. Wood writing in the popular magazine *Argosy*, contrasted the ability of the Chinese to withstand opium smoking whereas white middle-class consumers could not.

[V]ery many of these celestials and Indians are mentally and physically inferior, and they go on smoking year after year, and seem not very much the worse for it. It is your finer natures that suffer, deteriorate, and collapse. For these great and terrible is the ruin.[102]

In 1907 there were said to be two prosperous opium establishments in the East End, aimed exclusively at a white clientele and patronized by Englishmen or 'society women seeking a new sensation'. They were furnished in lavish style and entry was by means of a password.

This mix of racial fear and middle-class degeneration was to reach its height in the post First World War years, when it served to justify an extensive system of international control, as we will see in Chapter 7. Before the First World War, these fears about opium smoking in the UK were becoming linked to demands for more extensive and punitive control. The anti-opium forces were pushing for more stringent controls in the UK on smoking opium well before the war broke out. In July 1912 Theodore Taylor, Liberal MP for Radcliffe in Lancashire, presented a petition from the Chinese Gospel Mission in Liverpool, along with another 'influentially signed' one. At the Society's AGM in 1914 there were strong demands for a bill to be introduced into the House of Commons to prevent the spread of opium smoking from Chinese dens in the UK. Anti-opium organizations wanted an enquiry into opium smoking in the East End of London, Liverpool, Cardiff, and other ports. Taylor continued to stress the dangers of spread to the indigenous population.

[T]here will be a nemesis of the most terrible sort coming to us. This nemesis what is it? It is the talking hold of white people—people of our own flesh and blood—by this terrible vice of opium smoking.[103]

What was the reality of the practice so far as we can tell? It seems in many respects to have been more prosaic. How many 'dens' were there and where did smoking go on? Using the Pharmacy Acts to punish unqualified sales rarely happened as any stranger wanting to buy smoking opium would have been treated with suspicion. But seamens' lodging houses were licensed by the local authority, the London County

Council, which introduced compulsory licensing in 1909. Opium smoking could lead to withdrawal of a licence, much as allowing the smoking of cannabis on premises became a punishable criminal offence, albeit under a different set of laws, many decades later. But licensing was in practice often ignored and opium smoking went on in unlicensed premises. In 1912, twenty-nine Chinese houses in Lime-house were inspected early one morning, without warning. Eleven were licensed and eighteen unlicensed. In eleven of the unlicensed houses there was evidence of opium smoking; and the long delay in opening up in the other houses gave rise to suspicion that the same practice had been going on there. Police prosecution of unlicensed houses between 1910 and 1918 make it clear that almost any of the houses in the two streets in East London could have been used for opium smoking. The 'den' was a shifting entity, changing its location as often as the floating population of seamen in the area.

In fact, many of the more open-minded observers came to the conclusion that there was no such thing as an opium den, rather that it was a type of Chinese social club. The social investigator Walter Besant, who visited Pennyfields in the early 1900s, was surprised at what he found.

> We have read accounts of the dreadful place, have we not? Greatly to my disappointment, because when one goes to an opium den for the first time one expects a creeping of the flesh at least, the place was neither dreadful nor horrible.

Another writer in *The Times* saw opium smoking as less objectionable than overt drunkenness.

> We may call these places 'dens' for all that they are so clean and orderly and so little withdrawn from public gaze. We may deplore the injurious physical effects which follow over-use of the drug, however small the cases of definitely traceable injury may be either to the number of smokers or to the Chinese population. But we have to recognize first the universal human tendency to some form of indulgence in stimulants, and secondly the fact that all the 'dens' in these two streets together will not furnish from one month's end to another any such

spectacle of 'degradation' or rowdyism as may be seen nightly in almost any public house.

One way into this lost world of opium smoking is through oral history. It is now nearly a century since some of these 'den' descriptions were written, but there is some oral record of what people in the area thought. I interviewed one old man living in Limehouse some years ago. His view of what the Chinese did was rather different to the standard view. He had been a boy in the early 1900s and used to run errands for the Chinese seamen.

> You'd push a door open and you'd see them smoking…I used to be in number 11, and in that house there on the second floor we had one bed. But on the ground floor we had two, two beds. They were always there as they walked in, and as they fancied a piece of opium…In every house I have been in, there's been a bed or two. It was quite natural for the people who lived in that house…They're ordinary working people that come in here and have their pipe, because they're laid off from the shipping and they have their pleasure time in the Causeway as long as their money lasts.[104]

In his view, the idea that opium smoking was incompatible with hard work was wrong. Opium smoking was an aid to hard work, not a distraction from it, and smokers managed to combine their habit with a normal working existence.

> I've known them get up at eight, seven or eight in the morning, smoke opium twice, two periods of opium, and then go and do their duty, do their work, and they won't go to bed before eleven o' clock at night.

Another oral history project focused on a slightly later period. Annie Lai was an Englishwoman married to a Chinese shopkeeper in Limehouse in the 1920s, and by then, with the institution of more stringent postwar controls, life became difficult for opium smoking. But the trade was profitable and in the late 1920s and early 1930s opium retailed for two shillings for a small packet. Relations with the police could be tense but also accommodating.

> The local police were all right with us. Well they would use a little discretion with us—probably got a couple of bob now and again. From time

FEAR: DENS AND DEGENERATION

to time we'd get the word...But it was never the local police. It was the CID from Scotland Yard. But the local police had their duty so—they had to. So of course the word would go all around and everybody would be getting rid of everything...dope, the pipes.[105]

So it is clear that the actual practice of opium smoking was very different from the veneer of mystery and menace with which it became overlaid. But the symbolic and practical importance of that image was greater. The image of opium smoking both reflected and constructed a new view of drug use in society, a changing of culture. It also led, through the impact of the anti-opium agitation, to significant changes in international legal controls after the First World War as we will see in Chapter 7.

In the United States, there were similar racial fears about Chinese immigration and the connection with opium smoking. Initially Chinese immigration was welcomed—as part of the gold rush to California in the 1840s and 1850s. The Chinese moved into California and then spread out over the West to Oregon, Utah, Nevada, Idaho, Montana, Wyoming, and Texas. Most towns had a Chinatown where opium smoking went on. This, and the possible association of Chinese with prostitution, caused a change of heart. The Chinese were seen as potentially subverting American middle-class moral values. In the town of Deer Lodge, Montana, *The Deer Lodge New North-West* noted on 16 January 1880 that Deer Lodge did not possess an opera house, city government, or hurdy-gurdy house but it did have an opium den.[106] The same fears surfaced as in England—that respectable middle-class society would be subverted and in particular white women would be sucked in and their morals undermined. In 1882 a Chinese exclusion act was passed which reflected anti-immigrant fears, and by 1895 at least eighteen states and territories had passed anti-opium legislation. There was also union opposition to Chinese labour, as in the UK. In 1909 Congress approved a law 'An Act to prohibit the importation and use of opium for other than medicinal purposes'. This forbade the import of smoking opium by anyone and, significantly, drew the boundaries between (legitimate) medical use and (illegitimate) non-medical use around the issue of opium for smoking.

The fear of the Chinese as 'the other' and the racial dimension to responses to drug use was, if anything, greater in the USA than in the UK because of the ethnic diversity of the population. Cocaine use and blacks held particular fears for Southern society, expressing the fear that cocaine users might attack white society. One belief about cocaine was that it improved pistol marksmanships and also made blacks impervious to 0.32 calibre bullets. It is said to have caused southern police departments to switch to 0.38 calibre revolvers.[107] Such fears expressed the unease of white society rather than the reality of the drug's effects and also added a rationale to the ongoing repression of the minority group.

A major part of the fear of urban degeneration that marked the late nineteenth century and of which this fear of opium smoking was part, was the association with women. What Barry Milligan called the 'miscegenative dynamics of the opium den' was a key anxiety.[108] Dickens used this theme in *Edwin Drood* where the figure of the Englishwoman who smokes in the den is transformed by the activity.

> The woman has opium-smoked herself into a strange likeness of the Chinaman. His form of cheek, eye and temple, and his colour are repeated in her. (38)

That Englishwoman goes on to infect the Englishman John Jasper who smokes in the den.

> As he watches the spasmodic shoots and darts that break out of her face and limbs, like fitful lightning out of a dark sky, some contagion in them seizes upon him: insomuch that he has to withdraw himself to a lean armchair by the hearth—placed there, perhaps, for such emergencies— and to sit in it, holding tight, until he has got the better of this unclean spirit of imitation.

Jasper carries back the opium smoking habit to his cathedral town. He is the prototype of a character who became object of fascination for Victorian fiction—the respectable middle-class man who leads a second hidden life of uninhibited self-indulgence in the East End.

Later, in the period just after the First World War, the theme of opium smoking and degeneration of white women continued, albeit in rather different circumstances, in the Billie Carleton case of 1918–19. Billie, a popular success at the Haymarket Theatre, was found dead in bed in November 1918 after she had attended a victory ball at the Albert Hall. Cocaine was said to be to blame (it was actually veronal) but the lurid press exposés of the time also laid bare the limited opium smoking 'scene' and the place of white women in it. Opium smoking as well as cocaine was a 'smart' activity in certain demi-monde bohemian circles and the opium connection made perhaps more public impact than Billie's 'doping' with cocaine. The actress herself had been with a friend to Limehouse to smoke opium, but most of the activity took place in West End flats and opium smoking parties had been fashionable for several years before her death. At one, held in September 1918 in a flat off Piccadilly, Mrs Ada Ping You, Scottish wife of a Limehouse Chinese, prepared the opium. As she passed round the opium pipe, the five people present sprawled on the floor on cushions and pillows. 'The men divested themselves of their clothing and got into pyjamas, and the women into chiffon nightdresses. In that manner they seemed to prepare themselves for the orgy.'[109] These were 'dens of iniquity', with an 'opium orgy in night attire', and Mrs Ping You the 'High Priestess of Unholy Rites'. Opium smoking parties in the West End were the 'most disgusting orgies' where 'men and women...recline in a circle on soft cushions, and pass from hand to hand and mouth to mouth the opium pipe, from which they inhale the fumes of the drug and pass for a time into oblivion'. The case attracted huge publicity and the Chinese connection was translated into a 'Chinese Moriarty'—a Chinese 'Mr Big' who ran a network of dealing in smoking opium.

The harsher attitude towards drug use which this served to justify will be discussed in Chapter 7. The mix of women, racial minorities, and drugs was a heady combination, which drew on fears which were widespread at the turn of the century. How then did such fears affect alcohol—or tobacco? Women were again centre stage in fears about alcohol use but in a significantly different way. Alcohol played a key role in turn of the century degeneration fears; but the ways these were expressed—and for tobacco, which also played a role—were different, and contributed towards the different paths taken by the substances. A key divergence was the absence of a connection with racial minority use. For alcohol the major concern was with women's use and the impact this might have on what, in the terminology of the time, was called 'the future of the race'. Women as mothers and the impact of alcohol use on children was the focus.

The Victorians, and European theorists of insanity in general, believed in the idea of degeneration. Morel's theory of hereditary degeneration, mentioned in the previous chapter, was adopted by English psychiatrists. These believed in what was called the transmission of acquired characteristics through the generations. Thomas Clouston, for example, in his *Clinical lectures on Mental Diseases* (1883) gave great weight to the importance of hereditary transmission.

> The facts of nature compel the physician to see that the purely mental qualities and mental defects are transmissible from parent to child, and prepare him for the great part that heredity plays in psychological development and in mental disease. It has not yet been proved statistically whether the slope of a man's nose or the acuteness of his moral sense is the most apt to be transmitted to his children or grandchildren, but I am strongly of opinion that the latter will be found to be so.[110]

The idea relied on Lamarckian ideas that characteristics acquired by parents were passed on to their children—rather than a Darwinian position that change was the result of mutations either adapted to the environment or not.

A particular set of conditions stood out in these discussions; alcoholism was the most prominent among them. The nature of the hereditary transmission of alcoholism was a major subject of debate in the first decade of the twentieth century. Family histories were studied: the Jukes and the Kallikacks in America, the Jurkes in France, and the Phultains in England were characteristic in this type of investigation which dominated between 1860 and 1910. Many of the investigators were also temperance supporters. One widely quoted study was that of

R. Demme, who in 1885 published the results of a comparison of ten sets of sober parents and ten sets of alcoholic parents. The ten sober couples produced 61 children of whom seven died in infancy, two were mentally deficient, two were deformed, and the remaining fifty normal. In the remaining group of alcoholic families, the results were alarming. The ten families had produced nine normal and forty-nine abnormal offspring. The Swiss psychiatrist August Forel took these observations and moulded them into a theory of alcoholic degeneration called 'blastophoric degeneration'. He concluded that alcohol could affect the reproductive cells in both an acute and a chronic way. Intoxication at the time of conception resulted in what he called acute blastophoria of the offspring, yielding an increased number of children with epilepsy, imbeciles, and other abnormalities. Sir Victor Horsley and Mary Sturge in their investigation of *Alcohol and the Human Body* (1907) concluded that:

> The hygienic faults of parents are visited upon their children, if the latter survive the first few months of life, they are threatened with idiocy or epilepsy, or, still worse, are a little later on carried off by tuberculous meningitis or consumption.[111]

Horsley and Sturge also conducted experiments on the effect of alcohol. Cress wilted and kittens lost their ability to purr; the implications were alarming.

These ideas informed the debate on inebriety in European countries, and leading specialists in England such as Norman Kerr strongly promoted the idea of alcoholic heredity, in particular the transmission of the drink crave itself. The idea appeared in the report of the interdepartmental committee on physical deterioration in 1904, the major enquiry into the impact of 'race poisons' on the role of Britain as an imperial power.

There were counter arguments which came to a head in the 1890s. The British physician Sir G. Archdall Reid was a follower of August Weismann, who challenged the orthodox position on the transmission of acquired characteristics. Reid argued that characteristics acquired by the parents were not inherited by the child, and also went on to argue against legislative intervention in the form of alcohol control, treatment, or temperance. This was because alcohol could be a significant factor in eliminating those in society who were 'unfit'. Reid argued that alcohol 'is the cause of an evolutionary protective against itself. Drunkenness among the ancestry is the cause of temperance among the descendants.'[112] This explained why Western nations consumed alcohol and why colonial people seemed to suffer so much from its effects. This was not because of the role of imperialism or colonialism, but because these races had not developed a tolerance to alcohol in the way Europeans had. Societies, it was argued, should not prohibit alcohol because this would prevent the primitive and unfit from being eliminated. This was a eugenic argument.

When these ideas first burst into the inebriety world in the late 1890s they caused great controversy. Kerr and Reid debated the point, Reid attacking what he called 'The Temperance Fallacy'. Kerr's argument was that children drank because their parents drank. Reid denied this, declaring that children drank because they inherited the inborn constitution of mind which rendered drinking delightful to the parent. He was strongly opposed to any artificial intervention, apart from prohibition of child bearing by alcoholics. 'We have no more right to interfere with these men who do not directly injure the community than we have to interfere with men who eat to excess or who smoke or bicycle to excess.'[113]

The new 'eugenic' arguments criticized the concept of acquired deterioration, but continued the idea of hereditary alcoholic taint in other forms. But a severe shock to the degenerationist position came in 1910 with the publication of work by the statisticians Karl Pearson and Ethel Elderton at the Galton Laboratory for National Eugenics at University College London. These used statistics to examine the effects of parental alcoholism on the physique and abilities of their offspring. Their conclusions were startling. There was no discernible connection between parental alcoholism and mental defects in their children, or with children's intelligence. In fact the general health of the children of alcoholic parents appeared on the whole to be slightly better than that of the children of parents who were sober. This research had a considerable impact on ideas about degeneration, which underwent a decline before and during the First World War. The rediscovery of Mendelian genetics affected the study of inheritance and some of the evidence of degeneration was seen as harmless variations, while others had more specific causes. The increasing influence of the Freudian movement also hastened the end of degenerationist thought.

But while it lasted, this all-encompassing mode of explanation had focused attention on the alcohol consumption of women, the group which came to assume the identity of 'the other' in the case of this substance. The role of women and children came to the fore as a major part of the debates on degeneration and, as we will see later on, a focus on women continued over the years. The interdepartmental committee's report in 1904 commented that male consumption had not led to degeneration but 'if the mother as well as the father is given to drink, the progeny will deteriorate in every way, and the future of the race is imperilled'.[114]

It was because women had taken to drink, as well as men, that the outlook for the future was so dire. This is an enduring argument which we can revisit later on. The Society for the Study of Inebriety focused its concern on the role of women as mothers and on the importance of healthy children. In July 1903, for example, it held a meeting on the theme of inebriety in women and its influence on children's lives. The titles and topics of the papers tell it all—the psychology of the inebriate mother; the effects of female alcoholism on racial degeneration; inebriety in women and the overlaying of infants; and the restoration of the female inebriate. The Society's evidence to the physical deterioration committee continued the theme. Drinking females were responsible for miscarriages and also for the production of deformed and stunted children because the foetus could receive alcohol from its mother's circulatory system. The presence of alcohol in breast milk, destroying its nutritional value, was a further driver for physical deterioration. The Society, in its meetings and publications, most notably the views of fourteen experts gathered together in T. N. Kelynack's *The Drink Problem in its Medico-Sociological Aspects* (1907), stressed this line of argument.

The eminent specialist Mary Scharlieb, opening a discussion in 1907 on alcohol and the children of the nation, identified individual rather than the structural causes of infant mortality. 'The high death rate among English babies is not dependent on poverty alone.' These arguments were part of an agitation, publicized by the journalist G. R. Sims, also a member of the Society for the Study of Inebriety, which focused on the drinking habits of working-class women.[115] T. N. Kelynack summed up the position.

> Undoubtedly much of the high infant mortality is due to alcoholism, and conditions directly…or indirectly arising from this morbid condition. The wide spread prevalence of alcoholism among women, especially during the reproductive period of life, is one of the most important factors making for racial-decay.[116]

In February 1907 the first of a series of six articles by G. R. Sims, 'The Cry of the Children' was published. Sims maintained that children were being 'slowly murdered in the dram shop in their mother's arms'. Growing numbers of infants were being taken in their mother's arms into public houses where they were given drink to taste. He offered the slogans 'Out of the Dram Shop' and 'Back to the Breast'. The revelations were part of a campaign which led to the enactment of the 1908 Children's Act, one clause of which excluded children under fourteen from licensed premises where the sale and consumption of alcohol occurred. Children could still fetch drink for their parents provided this took place in a separated-off sales or jug and bottle department. The aim was to exclude 'the toddler from the tavern'.

The clause of the Act can be seen, as David Gutzke has pointed out, as part of the Edwardian response to disturbing social changes, reflecting upper and middle-class fears of an alien and threatening working-class culture, but also of women's changing role in society. It was women's greater freedom outside the home which evoked fear, together with the declining birth rate, marriage property rights, and suffrage demands. The psychiatrist Robert Jones expressed this unease. 'Women are now the companions of men in...industrial pursuits, and the freedom to work on equal terms with men has caused...the same depressing physical and mental influences...for which stimulants offer a temporary relief.'[117]

The degeneration debate and the Children's Act was one area where alcohol and tobacco came together. For the Act also prohibited the sale of tobacco products to children less than sixteen years of age. The much weaker movement against tobacco was also affected by the same ideas about national efficiency and degeneration. Weaker nations had suffered decline through smoking. By the time of the Boer War it was claimed that perhaps a third of the rejects from the army in Lancashire were due to 'smokers' heart' so the idea that youths and children should stop smoking became commonplace in anti-tobacco literature.[118]

In the years leading up to the First World War, fear had shaped responses to all the substances. In some respects the nature of that fear drew on similar concerns—the overarching concern about national and urban degeneration and the fear that a process of imperial decline was underway. All the substances were affected by this late Victorian and Edwardian obsession and increased regulation of one kind or another was the result. But the nature of degeneration and the ways in which the substances were affected were significantly different. It was opium which was associated with a different, perhaps alien, mode of consumption and with racial minority use. That racial minority also linked the issue with international patterns of consumption and with use by Chinese in China and the Far East as well as in the UK. It meant that a significant non-orthodox, non-medical area of consumption was defined and singled out. That pattern diverged from the fear associated with alcohol and tobacco. There, no racial minority was involved and smoking tobacco was rarely associated with smoking opium— Sherlock Holmes' use in *The Man with the Twisted Lip* is one of the few examples. Women and children's use and the implications for the future of the race were the main concerns and fears. After the turn of the century, the issue appeared to have been dealt with by the children's legislation: the decline of degenerationist theory gave the matter less urgency. Women and children and the connection with alcohol and tobacco did not have the same international ramifications as did opium use. Nevertheless, the role of women would resurface after the Second World War in relation to those two substances and also for tobacco use as well. In recent times it has been a major driver of policy.

6

Economics and Technology: The Role of Industry

A British official report published early in 2012 on the subject of drink 'units' argued that if the government worked too closely with industry, brewers, and shops, then there would be potential conflicts of interest. Behind this statement lay a long-standing postwar debate about what role 'industry' should play in policy, in particular for the legal substances, tobacco and alcohol. Public health campaigners in the present day are usually vehemently against the involvement of such economic interests in policymaking and we will be examining this recent constellation of anti-industry forces in Chapter 11. Industry is a short-hand term for the wider interplay of economic factors in the positioning of substances. Economic 'vested interests' and the allied role of technology and technical developments have played a significant role over a lengthy period in helping to determine their positioning. From at least the sixteenth century, trading interests drove the global expansion of substances. The American historian David Courtwright described that process succinctly 'The globalization of wine, spirits, tobacco, caffeine-bearing plants, opiates, cannabis, coca, and other drugs—was a deliberate, profit-driven process'.[119]

This chapter will examine the later history—from the eighteenth and nineteenth centuries—of the differential impact of economic and technical developments on the substances. Technical change and the growth of business interests for alcohol and tobacco in those centuries brought the development of mass markets and subsequent political influence. This was most marked for alcohol in Britain at least, in the period before the First World War. For the opiates and related substances such as cocaine, the picture was different. There, technical development—the isolation of the alkaloids and the development of the hypodermic syringe as the main means of drug delivery—brought a more restricted and medicalized market. The development of the pharmaceutical industry as a 'mass producer' came later than the alcohol developments and its influence on governments was different both through time and geography. This chapter will look at each of the substances in turn, rather than using a case study focused on one substance, to see how these factors played out.

Mass production came on the scene first for alcohol. Taking beer in Britain as an example, the eighteenth century saw important changes in production together with the types of product consumed. Private brewing declined and public brewing increased. Wholesalers and retailers both grew in proportion to the rest of production. There were already in mid century some large, highly capitalized businesses epitomized by the 'great brewers' of London. In 1748, the twelve largest of these accounted for over 40 per cent of London's output and by 1800 nearly 80 per cent. Calverts were the first to brew more than 50,000 barrels a year in 1748, Whitbreads first with 200,000 in 1796 and Barclays first with 300,000 in 1815. Historian John Burnett comments, 'This was industrialized brewing on a revolutionary scale, factory methods, technology and managerial skills applied to meet the demands of a mass market.'[120]

The dominance of the London brewers was based initially on a new product, 'porter', which was suitable for mass production. Before this, it had been the custom to order several beers and to mix them, something which caused much trouble for the publican, who had to go to three casks for a pint of liquor. Porter became a favourite in the London area—it was a heavy black beer brewed from brown malt. Peter Clark in his history of the alehouse talks about its significance as a mass product. 'Porter was one of the first truly mass-produced consumer items ever retailed in England, its success stemming from its strong appeal to publican and customer alike. It was potent, palatable, stable, long-lasting and cheaper than most of the strong beers and ales which it quickly displaced.'[121]

It also remained cheap. Economies of scale through mass production meant that prices remained stationary between the 1760s and the 1790s because of the expansion of the London breweries. Compared with general price trends, the cost of a pot of porter fell by a third.

The expansion into mass production and a mass product at first did not impact on breweries outside London. But from the mid nineteenth century, brewers in the Midlands, and in particular those in the town of Burton-on-Trent developed at a great rate. In the late eighteenth century, five major brewers had been located in close proximity along Burton High Street, producing 10,000 barrels of ale a year. Most of this was exported to the Baltic countries and the home trade expanded in the following century. There was a growing demand for lighter ales and after the 1840s the railways made national distribution of India export bitter possible. The rapid growth and profitability of this area of the industry were by words; by 1900 it was producing 10 per cent of British beer, or 3,500,000 barrels a year. The Bass brewing firm with Michael Thomas Bass at its head was the epitome of the new system. Its three breweries and 39 malt houses covered 145 acres; thirty-two steam engines and nine locomotives ran on twelve miles of private track. This was the biggest ale brewery in the world, producing a million barrels a year with a revenue of £1,000 a day for government coming from its annual turnover of £2,500,000. The firm's manager was reported to have produced his Bible to prove that the Bass hop store, six hundred feet long, was fifty feet longer than the reputed length of Noah's Ark.[122]

Later in the century further technical development took place with the rise of bottling and bottled beers. Such technical changes were important alongside the economics of the mass market. The rise of the London brewers had been underpinned by their use of the latest

technology, Boulton and Watt's steam engines, thermometers, hydrom-
eters, saccharometers, and attemperators. These enabled the production
of stable beer of reliable quality.[123] Later in the century, further technical
development and science made possible the production of fresher, 'running beers'. Refrigeration and also the application of Pasteur's theories
about fermentation and the development of pure yeasts to brewing
brought a better product. Pasteur's *Etudes sur la bière* published in 1876,
was not translated into English until 1879, but already English brewers
had begun to use the scientific approach and had appointed scientists to
oversee the brewing process.[124,125] In Ireland too, the firm of Guinness
also developed a mass market there using science as an aid.[126]

Spirits underwent a similar process of commodification and technical development which saw whisky emerge as a major new mass-
produced product. Spirit consumption rose in the third quarter of the
century, although it declined from the 1880s. Gin was still the most
popular spirit, but the commercialization and commodification of
Scotch whisky had begun in the 1820s. George Smith of Glenlivet built
up the largest commercial distillery in Scotland. The invention of the
patent Coffey still in 1830 gradually industrialized the production of the
spirit and aided the process. The most important development was the
blending of two distillates to produce a lighter and more flavoursome
spirit which appealed to English tastes. The development of blended
whiskies from the 1860s was led by firms such as James Buchanan, John
Walker, William Teacher, and John Dewar. These were marketed on a
mass scale by the wide merchants Gilbeys and by the Victoria Wine
Company. By the end of the century, whisky was the most popular
spirit in England, and was promoted by advertising and labels which
became household names.[127]

So mass production and the important role of technology and of science was important for the expansion of both beer and spirit consumption. Beer and spirits were exported but the amount of international
exchange of different types of liquor was limited. Lager beers were
developed in Germany from the 1840s and later in the Netherlands
(Heineken) and Denmark (Carlsberg) and some British restaurants

began to stock imported lager in the 1870s. But types of beer remained distinct. In the United States, German immigrants brought lager, their national type of beer, with them.

The brewing industry in England also developed a distinctive system of 'tied' public houses, which guaranteed the larger brewers established outlets. In 1817 almost half the licensed houses in London were tied. By the end of the century 75 per cent of licences were tied to brewers with an almost complete monopoly in some towns.[128] This was less a source of strength than of weakness for the industry. Whitbread's leasehold and freehold properties had been valued at £26,000 in the 1880s but were put at nearly £2 million by 1907. The Burton brewers also followed this line, paying prices which many considered to be 'insane'.[129] This made them vulnerable to the trade downturn in the early twentieth century as the shift to bottled beer and other leisure activities began. The large amount of 'tied' property also made the brewers sensitive to potential policy initiatives such as the compulsory reduction of licences. Off licences were given to licensed grocers, who sold wine and spirits to a more middle-class clientele. But the norm was the tied house, which gave the industry vertical integration. David Gutzke sums up how this affected the position of 'the trade'.'The closer link between brewer and retailer through the tied house system altered their activities as a pressure group, hurting the brewers' public image and threatening trade unity, but broadening the basis of public support, thereby weakening the Liberal zeal for prohibition and more generally retarding temperance reforms.'[130]

The national drink trade was of enormous financial importance to government at a time of expanding state activity. Liquor contributed to the British exchequer in two main ways: through duties on spirits, wine and beer and on the substances, such as malt, sugar, and hops, which went into making them; and duties on licences for making or selling alcoholic liquor. For most of the nineteenth century, taxes borne by alcohol provided a significant proportion of government revenue— well over 30 per cent, and even 43 per cent in the late 1870s. Revenue from Customs and Excise was also high—69 per cent in 1899–1900. But both were in decline from the early twentieth century—taxation had fallen to just over 14 per cent by the mid 1930s and Customs and Excise revenues to 34 per cent.[131]

The financial significance of alcohol to the exchequer is often still used as an argument to underline the political significance of drink. Even in the late eighteenth century, the brewers had had wealth and political influence behind the scenes, although this was at a local rather than a national level.[132] How that influence developed in the nineteenth century is more debatable. The 'drink question' did indeed become highly politicized in the nineteenth century in particular in the last quarter of the century. The Liberal Party, as we have seen, was allied to the temperance cause, although with waning enthusiasm from Liberal politicians before the First World War. Brewers and the Conservative Party began an alliance in the 1870s. In the 1895 general election when the Liberal Party was famously 'borne down on a torrent of gin and beer' after its attempt to introduce locally based prohibition, the drink trade had organized to secure a Liberal defeat. The Lancashire and Yorkshire brewers had decided the fate of forty constituencies, while in London, opposition was organized against every anti-Unionist candidate except the wine merchant, Mark Beaufoy.[133] But the Conservative and Unionist Party itself was uneasy at appearing to be too much in the pockets of the brewers. Temperance interests also exaggerated the influence of 'the trade' for their own ends. They discerned a conspiracy whereby Britain's Anglican governing elite sanctioned drink outlets to ensure that government revenues came from indirect taxation on working-class drinkers rather than direct property levies. The temperance reformers Joseph Rowntree and Arthur Sherwell, writing in 1899 about temperance and social reform, devoted a whole chapter to the menace of the drink trade, with its effect on local politics, municipal watch committees, as well as national politics.[134] It was this which led them to advocate state control of the drink trade. David Gutzke comments, 'According to this gloomy diagnosis, brewers had formed a huge state monopoly of formidable political power and commensurate wealth, which had thoroughly corrupted British republican institutions.'[135]

Historians have stressed that 'the trade' was in fact not the monolith of popular temperance propaganda but rather a much more disorganized set of organizations which found it difficult to unite on a common political agenda. Brewers and retailers really did not organize nationally much before the 1880s and the funds available for campaigning were much less than those raised for temperance. Records of firms in the Scottish whisky industry show that it was not until the 'People's budget' of 1909, which raised the excise duties on spirits, that those firms began to take an interest in being allied to the Conservative Party and in trying to influence shareholders and employees.[136] Changes in the drink trade in the 1890s had made the industry more of a publically accountable entity. Beginning in 1887, the large Burton and London breweries were floated on the stock exchange: the 1890s saw a surge of speculation about the fortunes of the industry with fierce competition, particularly in London, with the large brewers responding by a policy of purchasing public houses directly and also taking over the smaller breweries, often to gain control of their tied houses. The political implications of these changes, as John Greenaway has pointed out, were two fold. The leading breweries were overexposed in public house property and therefore sensitive to proposals for compulsory licence reduction. As public companies they were also accountable to a wider public. This meant that 'the trade' could pose as representative of a major legitimate public interest. Such changes caused alarm in temperance ranks and in the licensing controversies of 1904 and 1908, the issue of shareholders' influence was of concern. 167 peers and 129 MPs in 1904 had interests in brewing and distilling.[137] The 'beerocracy' was also enormously wealthy. The historian William Rubinstein's calculations showed that brewers formed one of the largest groups of all non-landed millionaires as represented by declared value of estates at death, even if they preferred to disguise the source of their wealth in published biographies.[138] Economic difficulties also brought the trade more into active politics, with declining consumption from the 1870s and a greater sense of crisis in the 1900s. The trade's interest in political influence came as its economic position was weakening.

Three key developments from economics and technology impacted on this substance and its position in this case study of British economic and technical development: the consolidation of producers and rationalization of production to feed a mass market; technical change which brought standardization and national distribution, a truly mass product—which remained a national rather than an international enterprise; and finally it brought political influence, albeit less significant than temperance interests maintained it was. The British case was not the model for all countries. In the Scandinavian countries, for example, there were state monopolies for the production and sale of alcohol, with the exception of Denmark and Sweden at the retail level, as we saw in Chapter 3, which had the Gothenburg System, where a local trust company was in charge of selling drink on a non-profit basis in order to discourage, not encourage drinking. The model was followed in some areas of Scotland but never took off in England, where mass production dominated.

At first sight, tobacco followed a similar path of business consolidation and mass production in the nineteenth century. But there were significant differences from alcohol—in the nature of the market; the political 'pull' of tobacco; and also the link to the retail trade.

The 1860s was the beginning of a time of growth for the tobacco industry. The process whereby it became characterized by the cigarette began at that time. Historian Howard Davies characterized the rise of what he calls 'the modern international cigarette'. First, it was manufactured from types of tobacco leaf whose species and method of curing both originated in the United States. Second, it was packaged and sold as a branded product using marketing methods whose earliest exponents were American firms. Third, it was a standardized product made using methods of mass production which originally became known as the American system of manufacture, and on a machine whose inventor was an American entrepreneur. 'In short, the modern international cigarette is an American invention.'[139] He identified four broad phases of development. In the last two decades of the nineteenth century, the industry moved from hand rolled to machine made products. American firms such as Allen and Ginter developed an export market in Europe for their colourfully packaged hand rolled cigarettes. These companies pioneered the growth of branded cigarettes in Britain and stimulated similar forms of production among local firms such as Players and Wills. To expand the market and replace the large numbers of women employed in hand rolling, some form of machine production was looked for. The most successful design was that patented by an American, James A. Bonsack, in 1881. But Allen and Ginter were reluctant to adopt mechanization when the reputation of their product had been built on hand rolling. European firms took the initiative and Cox is not totally correct in only emphasizing the US developments.

The first companies to use mechanized processes were the French tobacco monopoly and the British Bristol-based firm of W. D. and H. O. Wills. In Britain cigarettes had gained in popularity during the Crimean War and the new process of flue curing also dated from that period. Bonsack took his machine to Paris in 1883 and it was there that Harry Wills went over to inspect the machine in operation. His cousin Charles Hopkinson, a consultant engineer in Manchester, was called in to report. He concluded,

> The model with unpractised hands produced tolerable cigarettes, the defects that appeared were all such as can be rectified by skill in working the machine or in improvement in the machine. The rate of production was 8,000 per hour good and bad all counted. From this I infer that Strouse's statement of an actual production of 70,000 a day, which he offers to guarantee, on the iron machine, is really a sound working estimate, making allowance for starting, stopping and adjusting the machine.[140]

On 9 May 1883, an agreement was signed between Wills and the Bonsack company which included an exclusive right to the patent.

Wills was ahead of the first American tobacco manufacturer to install the machine for cigarette production. Several tobacco firms in the USA had shown interest in the machine, among them W. Duke and Sons of Durham, North Carolina. The firm experimented with the Bonsack in 1884 and in 1885, decided to bring it into full operation. James

Duke was the dynamic force in this company, creating new forms of industrial organization alongside mass production. He had begun to express interest in purchasing competitors in the late 1880s and at the turn of the century, created a new organization called a tobacco trust. In January 1890 he forced other major competitors to join this consortium, called the American Tobacco Company (ATC). This then acquired other companies, closing their plants and consolidating machinery, inventory, and products. The company had a national network to market and distribute products. There was also vertical consolidation of the business—as Duke developed extensive interests overseas in Canada and Australia, and also in Japan and China.[141]

The way in which this was done was novel. A problem of excess capacity built up during the 1880s and many of the leading American and British firms sent representatives round the world to seek orders for their products. ATC products flooded into the markets of Japan and China—annual exports in the 1890s of ATC cigarettes increased from 300 million to over one billion. But then there was a problem. Competition from local tobacco firms, and the tendency for local tariffs to rise to keep out the foreign imported cigarette, meant that from 1894 ATC began to transfer production directly into these foreign markets through partnership arrangements or direct acquisition. This was an American tactic: British firms who moved into foreign markets did so on the basis of exports not of direct acquisition, or even of licensing before 1900.

It was when Duke tried to extend this tactic of acquisition to Britain in the early 1900s that trouble occurred. Only one British company was prepared to accept Duke's offer of merger and the others, including Wills and Players, banded together to fight off Duke's advances through the formation of the Imperial Tobacco Company. After a 'tobacco war' lasting twelve months, a truce was agreed. ATC and Imperial were each to confine their activities to their respective national markets. All their foreign investments and export trade were transferred to a British registered joint venture called the British-American Tobacco Company (BAT Co), ATC's contribution of international assets to this new company allowed the American company to claim two thirds of the initial equity stake, although the company's headquarters were located in London rather than New York. James Duke even moved to London to enable his active management at the London HQ.

This monopoly agreement only lasted until the end of the First World War. America was committed to freeing business up, not tying it down in restrictive practices. The Sherman anti-trust act showed the opposition of US government to this sort of business arrangement and insisted on the dismemberment of the trust. In 1911 the government ordered it to be dissolved. ATC had to dispose of its holding in the BAT Co leaving Imperial as the leading minority shareholder. BAT Co had emerged by the end of the war as a British controlled firm. The decision also created a group of independent firms now free to expand overseas and to engage in competition with BAT Co. Four successor manufacturers emerged—Liggett and Myers, R. J. Reynolds, Lorillard, and a reformed ATC. These formed an oligopoly who struggled for shares in the US market while BAT Co strengthened its international position by making investments in the South American markets of Argentina and Brazil.

During these years of rapid expansion and organizational change, the position of the cigarette remained marginal relative to overall tobacco consumption. The popularity of cigarette smoking had spread during the 1890s but by 1901 cigarettes still accounted for only fourteen and a half per cent of UK consumption of all tobacco goods. Price was a factor—cigarettes selling at five for 1d were 50 per cent dearer to the smoker than medium-priced packet tobaccos. But this situation was changing and the significance of the price differential was steadily reduced over time, in particular as the smoker's outlay for a given weight of tobacco became a proportionately smaller part of his expenditures.[142] The historian Bernard Alford shows how cigarette consumption rose much faster than total tobacco consumption, a process driven by changing tastes. Wills dominated the market for cigarettes and their best-selling cigarette was the Woodbine. In 1907, 5,000 million Woodbines were smoked, far exceeding the combined consumption of all the other Imperial cigarette brands, and six times more than the next largest selling brand, Player's Medium. In 1919, cigarette sales overtook the sales of all other tobacco products in the UK; by this time Imperial had secured a virtual monopoly of UK cigarette production. The ways in which this market expanded in the 1920s and 1930s will be considered in Chapter 8. The rise of mass production brought a change in the role of the retailer. There were parallels here with outlets for drink, although the relationship to the producer was different. Prior to mass production the retailer had acted as some kind of guarantor of quality, relying on skills of selection, mixing, and preparation of tobacco. But mass production took away this role and brought branded or proprietary products centre stage. There were two different types of tobacco dealers—those licensed to deal in a range of tobacco and those who only sold pre-packaged goods in kiosks. The licensed trade remained important, with half a million licensed dealers even in the 1930s, one of the largest retail trade associations.[143] But, unlike drink, they were not 'tied' to the producer. The cheap price of the licence meant that the trade stayed open, with a range of traders, including the pharmacies mentioned in Chapter 4. Imperial did not need vertical integration and did not need to own distribution outlets, because of the cultural dominance it secured over them.[144]

On the surface then, there was much which was similar between tobacco and alcohol in terms of the role of economics and technology. The consolidation and integration of production and distribution to a mass market of a mass-produced mechanized product, with control of retailing—for tobacco—all recall the nineteenth-century drink story. The 'rise of the cigarette' came later, in the first half of the twentieth century, than the popularity of the mass-produced drinks. But there were also other significant differences. The tobacco firms, in the UK at least, did not at this stage, have the political influence of the brewers and in the USA the state actively forced the break up of the tobacco trust arrangement. The tobacco market, and in particular, the cigarette market, was an international one at the same time as it became a mass-produced one. The story of expansion, despite the existence of national cigarette industries and state monopolies like the one in France, was also a study in globalization.

China was one country where expansion of cigarette distribution was rapid during and after the First World War. Significantly, this took place at a time when the opium trade was in decline. Cigarettes were imported into China for the first time in the 1890s and cigarette smoking spread to all classes at a time when the anti-opium movement was spreading and the trade between India and China in opium was drawing to a close, as we saw in Chapter 3. Cigarettes were smoked by all classes after the spread of the anti-opium movement. British American Tobacco's greatest success was in China in the early twentieth century, where it created an integrated system of mass production and distribution. The historian Frank Dikotter points out that the US government was an opponent of opium sales, in which it had no financial stake, but gave no opposition to the growing cigarette industry from which it stood to gain fiscally.[145]

The different positioning of tobacco and opium at the beginning of the twentieth century through economic expansion brings us to the case of drugs and of opium and coca, later cocaine, in particular. Here we can outline a different trajectory although some of the elements of the story, new products, mechanized production, the rise of a consolidated industry, were similar. But they led to a different type of market.

For drugs, the key initial technical development was the isolation of the alkaloids of opium. The use of the active principle to produce a more powerful and standardized product was an important development at a time when adulteration of drugs and variable quality was an issue of concern. The isolation of morphine came early in the nineteenth century. Three chemists and pharmacists shared the responsibility. In 1803, Derosne, a French manufacturing chemist, produced a salt which he called his 'sel narcotique de Derosne', a substance later known as narcotine but also containing some morphine. A year later, Armand Seguin read a paper before the Institut de France in which he described his isolation of the active principle of opium. This communication 'Sur l'opium' was not published until 1814. Meanwhile, Frederick

William Serturner, a pharmacist of Einbeck in Hanover, working on Derosne's salt, had investigated the composition of opium more accurately. Isolating a white crystalline substance, which he found to be more powerful than opium, he called the new substance 'morphium', after Morpheus, the god of sleep. The *Journal der Pharmazie* published some details of this work in the early 1800s although the significance of the work was not appreciated until 1816. In 1831 the Institut de France awarded him a substantial prize for 'having opened the way to important medical discoveries by his isolation of morphine and his exposition of its character'.[146]

The discovery of the alkaloid was part of the growth of toxicology as a science and a general systematization of remedies. Quinine, caffeine, and strychnine were all isolated shortly after morphine. Other alkaloids of opium were also discovered—narceine by Pelletier in 1832 and codeine by Robiquet in 1821. Robiquet made the discovery while examining a new process for extracting morphine suggested by Dr William Gregory of Edinburgh. Morphine first became known in Britain in the 1820s and was sometimes called 'morphium'.

Technical discovery was allied with production and the alkaloid was manufactured on a commercial scale quite early on. It was produced by Thomas Morson, later one of the founders of the Pharmaceutical Society and one of its presidents. Morson had trained initially as a surgeon in Paris, where much of the 'new knowledge' lay, and had picked up his pharmaceutical expertise there. On his return to England, he took over a pharmaceutical business in Farringdon Street in London. Morphine and other drugs were produced in the parlour behind the shop. Morson's first commercial morphine was produced in 1821, at about the same time that the firm of Merck in Darmstadt in Germany also began to produce wholesale morphine. A price list of the time shows the English variety sold at eighteen shillings a drachm, with the acetate and sulphate selling at the same rate.

Another company also came into the morphia business in the 1830s. Macfarlan and Company of Edinburgh began to manufacture the alkaloid in the early 1830s, when Dr William Gregory, whose father James

Gregory had produced an opium based patent medicine, Gregory's Powder, invented a process for the manufacture of the muriate of morphia. Opium came to Edinburgh from the London drug houses and Macfarlan's returned the muriate. The manufactured drug was brown, like opium, and formed a brown solution. Later on, when Macfarlan's developed a purer white substance, they had difficulty in persuading purchasers to accept it. In these early days, different morphine products were used-including the muriate, hydrochloride and acetate of morphia; the first two later became established as standard. Later on preparations such as bromide of morphine, bimeconate, morphine sulphate, and morphine tartrate also came onto the market.

The drug was recommended in the text books for almost as many conditions as opium. It seems, from looking at the medical journals and also case histories, that it was in enthusiastic use from the 1830s and 1840s. It found a place in the London Pharmacopoeia in 1836. By the end of the 1830s, medical men were discussing in some detail the dose they preferred. Case notes show that in King's College Hospital in London, morphia was in routine use as early as 1840, mostly for sleeplessness.

Alongside dosage, another issue discussed was the form in which the drug should be administered, and out of this came the next significant technical development. Morphia was never administered solely by mouth. For example, there were morphia suppositories—Dr Simpson's Morphia Suppositories, made of morphia and sugar of milk, dipped into white wax and lard plaster melted together were made by Duncan and Flockhart of Edinburgh. One surgeon was horrified to find that his dog had swallowed a whole batch which had been made with mutton fat. The drug was also used by rubbing on the skin, known as endermic use. This was already in practice for opium. Michael Ward, physician to the Manchester Infirmary, published *Facts Establishing the Efficacy of the Opiate Friction* in 1809 and had pointed out that opium through the skin had a different effect to that administered by mouth. For the endermic method, a section of skin would be removed, usually by blistering and the powdered drug would be applied directly; this was a popular mode for morphine. A chemist's prescription book for Islington in North London, where details of practice were recorded, shows that Mr Hanley was prescribed morphine hydrochloride in liquid form in 1865, also to be absorbed through the skin. He was to 'dip a little bit of soft lint into the lotion and lay it upon the most painful part occasionally'.[147]

The development of hypodermic administration was the technical development which replaced these cruder attempts to produce a more immediate drug effect. Hypodermic injection was a technical innovation of the mid nineteenth century, but intravenous administration had a longer history. Drugs had been injected into both animals and humans since at least the seventeenth century. At the end of the eighteenth century, the new practice of inoculation, a precursor of vaccination, revived interest in the method. Dr Lafargue of St Emilion wrote a series of letters and papers in the 1830s in which he described his method for the inoculation of morphine. The point of a surgeon's lancet was dipped into a solution of morphine, then inserted horizontally beneath the epidermis and allowed to remain there for a few seconds. Larfargue's researches developed in a different direction and in the 1840s, he was proposing that medicated pellets be implanted with a darning needle.

As with the isolation of morphine, three men take credit for the development of the hypodermic method. These were Dr Rynd of Dublin, Dr Alexander Wood of Edinburgh, and Dr Charles Hunter, a house surgeon at St George's Hospital in London. Rynd, who worked at the Meath Hospital and County Infirmary in Dublin in the 1840s, described how he had cured a female patient of neuralgia by introducing a solution of fifteen grains of acetate of morphine by four punctures of 'an instrument made for the purpose'. The patient recovered, as did others treated in the same way. Ten years later, Alexander Wood, apparently unaware of Rynd's earlier publication, described his own method of treating neuralgia. He had made several attempts to introduce morphia through punctured needles, and, in 1853, 'I procured one of those elegant little syringes constructed for the purpose by Mr Ferguson of

Giltspur Street, London'. An elderly lady suffering from neuralgia was the guinea pig and recovered well; Wood published papers in the 1850s which publicized the method.

Dr Charles Hunter's use of the new method revealed its true potential. Hunter initially followed Wood in using the method as a local means of treating disease. But the site became infected and he was forced to inject elsewhere, soon realizing that the results were just as good. He advocated the 'general therapeutic effect' of hypodermic medication, in opposition to the localized influence which Wood and others believed in. What he called his 'ipodermic' (later hypodermic) method was a matter of sustained and acrimonious debate between the two men. Wood had described a general effect in a paper published in 1855, but later clung to the idea that it was a localized means of treating a local infection. The controversy created such interest that the Royal Medical and Chirurgical Society, to which Hunter had read a paper on the topic in 1865, appointed a committee to look into the question of hypodermic medication. Its report was published in 1867 and came down strongly on the side of Hunter. It concluded that 'no difference had been observed in the effects of a drug subcutaneously injected, whether it be introduced near to, or at a distance from the part affected'.

This endorsement unleashed a process often since seen in the drugs arena—a period of unquestioning enthusiasm for a new scientific development or new drug apparently without problems in its administration. Hunter proposed a wide range of uses for morphia— melancholia, mania, and delirium tremens. It was also useful for chorea, puerperal convulsions, peritonitis, ague, uterine pain, tetanus, rheumatism, and incurable diseases such as cancer. Dr Francis Anstie, Editor of *The Practitioner* was particularly enthusiastic. Anstie edified the journal from its foundation in 1868 and was determined to promote new and more exact scientific remedies for disease. His warmest praise was reserved in the early years of the journal for the hypodermic method and for its use with morphia. His 1868 article 'The hypodermic injection of remedies' accepted the method unquestioningly...of *danger* he wrote, there is *absolutely none*...The advantages of the hypodermic injection of morphia over its administration by the mouth are immense...the majority of the unpleasant symptoms which opiates can produce are entirely absent...it is certainly the fact that there is far less tendency with hypodermic than with gastric medication to rapid and large increase of the dose, when morphia is used for a long time together.[148]

The promotion of hypodermic morphia was part of the process of establishment of medical expertise at the expense of non-medical, non-specific remedies such as opium—whose use was usually denigrated when the use of morphia was advanced.

Gradually, however, the first warnings about the drug began to appear. Clifford Allbutt, later Regius Professor of Physic at Cambridge had initially been an enthusiast, and had used hypodermic morphine to treat heart disease where opium was forbidden. But in 1870 he expressed doubt in the pages of *The Practitioner*. Nine of his patients seemed as far from cure as ever despite their prolonged use of morphia.

Gradually...the conviction began to force itself upon my notice, that injections of morphia, though free from the ordinary evils of opium eating, might, nevertheless, create the same artificial want and gain credit for assuaging a restlessness and depression of which it was itself the cause.[149]

Allbutt's warning did not lead to immediate change in prescribing, and doctors still wrote enthusiastically to the medical journals about the good results they obtained with the drug.

But there was a dawning realization that morphine injections on a repeated basis could have attendant dangers. Reports of the usefulness of the method were tinged with wariness in particular as details of the abuse of the drug and the method in Europe and the United States began to filter through. In Chapter 4 we looked at how theories of inebriety and addiction began to be applied in many countries before the First World War and how morphine addiction was part of this process. Dr H. H. Kane of New York published in 1880 his book *The Hypodermic Injection of Morphia: Its History, Advantages and Dangers* based on British as well as American case histories and there was a more general discussion in public life of the place of morphia. In the House of Commons, the Conservative politician Lord Randolph Churchill, compared Gladstone's oratory on Home Rule to 'the taking of morphia! The sensations...are transcendent; but the recovery is bitter beyond all experience'.

Here was a process of technical innovation and industrial production which had led to a more restricted market. Even before the warnings about addiction, hypodermic morphine had been a more restricted and medicalized drug than over-the-counter opium. Preparations containing more than 1 per cent opium fell within the Pharmacy Act of 1868 and so had to be sold by a qualified pharmacist. In the 1908 Act they were moved into the more restrictive Part 1 of the poisons schedule. Control was not that stringent however. Even a doctor's prescription remained the property of the patient and could be redispensed at will and there was growing concern about this before the First World War.

Despite medical concern, numbers of morphine addicts appear to have been small, although the sources for this are difficult to assess. There are no figures for 'home consumption' of opium or morphine after duty was abolished in 1860. Morphine was not separately incorporated into trade statistics until 1911. There was a widening gap after 1860 between imports and exports which suggests that some of the imported drug was being used to make morphine; the best Turkish opium would yield around 10 per cent morphine. Yet how much morphine the firms of Morson and Son, J. F. Macfarlan, and T. and H. Smith in Edinburgh were producing and exporting is uncertain. The fears about morphine addiction also may have been the profession myopically exaggerating the dimensions of a problem it had helped to create. Certainly some of the use of hypodermic morphine prescriptions would have come to light through dispensing by pharmacists. The poisons register for an Eastbourne pharmacists practice giving details of transactions under the Pharmacy Act in the 1880s and early 1890s shows entries for morphia lozenges for cough but only one entry in a six-year period between 1887 and 1893 for sol.morph.hypo or hypodermic morphia.[150] Small numbers were admitted for treatment, about two a year taking morphia to the Dalrymple Home at Rickmansworth—but these would have been self-referred, not forced into treatment. The gender divide tended to the male rather than the female, despite the concern about women addicts and morphine tea parties.

Such conclusions are at variance with those reached on the basis of US evidence by the American historian David Courtwright, who generally supports what doctors were saying was the case—that women were the problem. But Courtwright is using figures for the import of medicinal opium, which presumably cover both opium and morphine. The mass market in both countries was for opium not for morphine, where more restricted access became the norm. However, in Britain, the official texts did not call the drug 'prescription only' until the 1930s.[151] Again there seem to be differences between Britain and the USA but there is little evidence that there was a rising epidemic of women morphine injectors.

Cocaine, the alkaloid isolated from the coca leaf, passed through a similar process. In 1855 Friedrich Gaedcke had produced from the distillate of the dry residue of an extract of coca a crystalline sublimate he called 'Erythroxylon'. But it was Albert Niemann of Gottingen who isolated pure cocaine from leaves which had been brought to Europe. In 1862, Wilhelm Lossen published its chemical formula and the isolation of other coca alkaloids followed later in the century.[152]

Initial enthusiasm was stimulated by the discovery by Carl Koller, Freud's collaborator, of its anaesthetic properties, in particular for eye surgery. Cocaine became a wonder drug. There were sixty-seven separate articles about it in the first 1885 volume of the *British Medical Journal*. Its use as a local anaesthetic in operations on the vagina and urethra, in dentistry, ophthalmic surgery, vaccination, operations on the nose and larynx, vomiting, mammary abscess, cancer, scalds, circumcision, neuralgia, hay fever, gangrene, nymphomania, sea sickness—there seemed to be no end to the possibilities. Patent medicines or wines based on coca or cocaine also brought the drug to a mass market.

In the United States and in Britain, concerns about addiction eventually brought more restrictive controls. Control of Food and Drug labelling in the States in 1906 required acknowledgement of the presence of cocaine in wines, several of which either withdrew from the market or modified their formula to exclude coca or cocaine at that time.[153] There was also a growing medical backlash against cocaine even though it remained an important local anaesthetic.

Cocaine and hypodermic morphine, although the product of technological change, did not become mass consumer products in the way in which alcohol and cigarettes did. But their isolation and development represented an important stage in the emergence of the pharmaceutical industry as a key player in both national and international affairs. In the USA Parke Davis manufactured cocaine and the leading company in Europe for the drug was Merck of Darmstadt. They had begun cocaine production using Peruvian coca leaves in 1862. In Germany alone at least thirteen pharmaceutical companies diversified into cocaine in the peak of enthusiasm of the 1880s. But Merck's product was recognized as superior. The industry remained fragmented before the First World War, however, and cocaine was never a primary product for the firms involved, including Merck. Richard Friman concludes that the firm was anything but a cohesive force in the years before 1914.[154]

So economics and technology had played a major role in shaping the futures of the three sets of substances. Technological change affected all three, as did the rise of different business and manufacturing models in tandem with industrial societies. For alcohol and for cigarettes this meant a mass product for a mass market; for drugs, the product was for a more restricted and medicalized market. Trading interests also operated to detach drugs from mainstream culture, as the Indo Chinese opium trade, which had supplied China, declined in the early twentieth century and tobacco consumption and cigarettes developed a mass market there. But the role of industry was important for drugs and there were major changes in the way in which the pharmaceutical industry was organized and its influence felt. The impact of that industry came at the international level during the First World War in ways which set the substances on their different paths. We turn to international ramifications in the next chapter.

7
Internationalism and War

On 24 July 1906, Bishop Brent of the Philippines wrote to the American President, Theodore Roosevelt,

My Dear Mr President,

I am going to make bold to suggest that which I venture to think might be fruitful of great good if you can see your way to initiating the movement. It is this: Recently, as of course you are aware, the question of England's share in the opium traffic has been reopened in official circles in the old country. My experience on the Philippine opium investigating committee leads me to believe that the problem is of sufficient merit to warrant an endeavour to secure international action. From the earliest days of our diplomatic relations with the East the course of the United States of America has been so manifestly high in relation to the traffic in opium that it seems to me almost our duty, now we have the responsibility of actually handling the matter in our own possessions, to promote some movement that would gather in its embrace representatives from all countries where the traffic in and use of opium is a matter of moment.

Why could we not hope to have an investigation on the basis of science as well as of practical observation of actual conditions, in which England, France, Holland, China, and Japan should take part with ourselves? The sole hope for the Chinese is in concerted action. As a side issue, but as a consideration that would in my mind enhance the value of the movement, it would tend to unify in some measure nations that are oriental either by nature or through the possession of dependencies in the Orient. Nothing tends to promote peace more than a common aim.[155]

Brent's letter was the portent of later international control of opiates and allied drugs. It leads us into the next crucial factor which has impacted differently on the substances; international agendas and the impact of war. The opiates and cocaine became subject to a system of international control just after the First World War, which grew out of concern about opium use in the Far East, but was also the result of US trade and strategic objectives in that area. This became a worldwide system, way beyond its original intention, because of the strategies adopted by pharmaceutical companies and the impact of the war. Pharmaceutical companies and their national governments argued for a more widespread control system before the war, in part because of concern about the spread of cocaine in the colonies, but also because the companies thought that there would never be global agreement on this. The delay ultimately brought a greater degree of control. Alcohol has had no such global restrictions placed on it, and control was limited in the same period to a regional system which just covered Africa. For tobacco, the idea of internationalism came on the agenda much later and in line with public health objectives, as we will see in Chapter 9. The World Health Organization's Framework Convention on Tobacco Control (adopted in 2003) now embodies the global focus of the anti-tobacco movement of the second half of the twentieth century.

This chapter argues that the First World War was crucial for the positioning of substances. A combination of international influences and war resulted in very different outcomes for drugs and for alcohol, while tobacco was simply off the international agenda at that time. War led to concerns about drug use, including cocaine dealing in the West End of London by troops on leave. The peace treaty brought into operation a system of international control, which has helped shape national systems ever since. This was not the outcome of national situations, but rather the outgrowth of pre-war colonial rivalries, overlain with US imperialist ambitions in the Far East. As noted earlier, what had been intended to be just a Far Eastern control system became, almost by accident, a worldwide system. It was this system which, again almost accidentally, first brought cannabis under stringent restriction in the 1920s.

The president did endorse Brent's idea, perhaps surprisingly, as the bishop was a relatively young man, in his early forties, only in the post for five years, and in charge of a diocese where there were few Protestants and few votes. The letter eventually went to the State Department from where it started two and a half years of diplomatic correspondence which led to the meeting of the Shanghai Opium Commission in 1909. Standing back at this stage and placing these events in context, Brent's stance, and the support it gained from international anti-opium interests, was part of a broader move to internationalism in both health and moral matters in the nineteenth century. The beginning of international health cooperation (that is, cooperation between two or more states) is traditionally located in the series of international sanitary conferences held between 1851 and 1903.[156,157,158] Even earlier, from 1815, regulations about quarantine shifted towards a concern for public health rather than trade.[159] The spread of epidemic diseases, especially cholera and yellow fever, was an important motive force. The two cholera pandemics that engulfed Europe between 1830 and 1847 were facilitated by the increased movement of goods and people between east and west that accompanied developments in international commerce: steamships, rail, and later the construction of the Suez Canal. The long-established response to epidemic disease, such as the plague, was to close ports and impose quarantine, but that proved difficult to sustain in the age of international commerce. Quarantine measures and disruption to shipping served to undermine the maritime economies of nations like Britain and France, whereas the speed of steamships meant that people and goods would have disembarked before a disease declared itself. The international sanitary conferences emerged as a mechanism for responding to the political and economic threats which a new epidemic disease such as cholera posed to the European powers.

Economic and imperialist conflicts surfaced at regular intervals throughout the conferences convened between the 1850s and 1903. The conventions and regulations that emerged from the majority of these conferences were never successfully ratified by participating governments. But in 1903 a conference held in Paris produced what Goodman describes as the 'first effective convention'. The 1903 convention formed the basis of the regulations governing quarantine on land and sea until the Second World War. Representatives of twenty governments including the USA, Egypt, Persia, and Brazil, as well as European nations, recommended the establishment of an International Office of Public Health. The Office International d'Hygiène Publique (OIHP) was established in 1907. It was based in Paris but maintained close communication with the regional sanitary councils and the health authorities in various countries. The primary function of the OIHP was the collation and dissemination of epidemiological intelligence. Governments were obliged to inform the office of the steps being taken to implement the sanitary conventions and the office could suggest modifications. The OIHP's coordination through regional councils and its focus on the health authorities of states prefigured the organizational emphasis of later bodies such as the WHO. The establishment of the OIHP marked the transition from the era of international conventions to that of permanent international health organizations, of which the Pan American Sanitary Bureau (PASB) was the first in 1903.

The development signalled by the emergence of the first international health organizations was part of a broader movement toward international cooperation, which had been growing in range and complexity throughout the nineteenth century. It is here that health and moral movements begin to overlap. The century from the Congress of Vienna (1815) to the outbreak of war in 1914 saw the emergence of wide-ranging international cooperation in many areas: law, economics, labour, religious, and intellectual movements, social and welfare organizations and humanitarian causes. There were nearly 3,000 international gatherings in this period and the creation of more than 450 private or non-governmental international organizations and over thirty governmental ones. Developments in transport and communication facilitated this level of international activity, and national governments vied for the patronage of international conferences.

Developments that can be considered as having a health dimension can be broken down into two fields: intellectual cooperation and consensus in science and social, religious, and humanitarian movements. At the close of the century the momentum for cooperation between non-state actors, and later between states, focused on the exchange of information, and represented the first moves towards an international vocabulary (standards, classification) in medicine and science. The social, religious, and humanitarian movements that emerged in the nineteenth century were more complex and diverse in their development. Many were characterized by popular and even mass support but there was also the pattern of conferences leading to more permanent committees or organizations. A burgeoning middle class and the spread of missionary activities supported many of the activities, whereas the shared experience of industrialization and urbanization spawned common social problems across a number of states. The first of four International Congresses of Charities, Correction and Philanthropy met in Brussels in 1865. These were followed in 1869 by a new series of international congresses on public and private charity that met at irregular intervals up to 1914.

A number of international 'single issue' reform movements also came to the fore, a development seen as early as 1840 with the International Anti-Slavery Conference and later the International Committee of the Red Cross (1864). In the health and welfare field these associations could be popular in orientation or focused on specialist expertise. Some mingled activism and science; one example was the international Central Bureau for the Campaign against Tuberculosis (1902), which emerged from a series of international conferences dating back to the 1860s. Movements against the African slave trade, the white slave traffic, and the peace and quarantine movements also paralleled the anti-opium story. The pattern was one of initial activity by non-state actors in the international arena, leading to greater intergovernmental involvement. For example, the policing conventions around the 'white slave trade', stemmed from the 1899 International Bureau for the Suppression of Traffic in Women and Children. The moves around opium leading to formal organizations also emanated from similar moral and internationalist concerns.

Brent's letter came at a propitious time and an interlocking sequence of events caused the initiative to gain momentum. The Opium War of 1840–2 and subsequent conflict in the 1850s between Britain and China had ended in China's defeat and laid the country open to foreign trade and missionaries. The standard image of these wars is of Britain forcing opium on a reluctant China. But recently historians have argued that the political significance of the war for later Chinese nationalism as 'imperialist aggression' has tended to downplay or ignore other significant contextual factors. For example, there was already growing demand and use of opium in China; it was cultivated widely by the Chinese themselves as a domestic drug; China's economic difficulties may not have been caused by the outflow of silver or the importation of opium. And finally, internal court politics had much to do with the abrupt change towards an official policy of prohibition, which in its turn led to the despatch of Commissioner Lin to Guangdong to bring all opium imports to a halt—the famous move which led directly to the first war.[160] One of the most recent revisionist histories, by Julia Lovell, has pointed to the long afterlife of the war as symbol. Chinese governments after Tiananmen Square in 1989 adroitly used the 'century of national humiliation' to bolster Communist Party authority and the right to rule in order to persuade the people that the Party was the sole defence against a West that had conspired since the nineteenth century to sabotage China.[161]

By the end of the nineteenth century and the early years of the twentieth, a movement for change in the trade was gaining momentum. The report of a Royal Commission on Opium published in 1895 had taken a different, more tolerant view of opium use. Primarily focused on the role of opium in India, it accepted the continuing importance of the drug as an accepted part of Indian culture. It concluded:

> opium is extensively used for non-medical and quasi medical purposes, in some cases with benefit, and for the most part without injurious consequences. The non-medical uses are so interwoven with the medical

uses that it would not be practicable to draw a distinction between them in the distribution and sale of the drug.[162]

In the early twentieth century, the position on opium altered. The Indo Chinese trade was in decline because Chinese domestic production of opium was rising. As early as 1885, China was probably producing at least twice as much opium as she was importing and twenty years later this figure had risen to four times as much.[163] Alongside this went a change in the balance of anti-opium forces in both Britain and China. In Britain, anti-opium political muscle was given weight by the return of a Liberal government in 1906 for which opium was a potent political symbol. The Indian opium monopoly, with its substantial government involvement (it collected opium and sold it to wholesalers) could no longer be so easily defended. In China, too, opium was a symbol in the Chinese reform movement. Chinese students returning from Japan began to call for reform after observing the operation of a government monopoly there and in Formosa, and its effect in helping reduce opium smoking. After the Boxer Rebellion, the Qing Dynasty issued an edict in 1906 requiring the cessation of opium cultivation over a ten year period and instituting licences for smokers based on the model used in Formosa.[164]

Increased domestic control was accompanied by significant activity on the foreign policy scene. Civil servants in the British Foreign Office were professional cynics, in particular about American motives—but they did agree to open up negotiations with the Chinese about the ending of the Indo-Chinese trade. At the same time as Bishop Brent was urging the State Department to action, negotiations between Britain and China led to an agreement that the British government would reduce Indian opium exports by 10 per cent a year, provided the Chinese reduced domestic production by the same amount. The British were concerned that the Chinese might simply increase their own production to compensate for the loss of Indian opium. So they insisted on independent verification of Chinese progress. Three years after the initial agreement, a London designated inspector would be allowed unlimited access to the interior. If the initial efforts were seen to be a success, then both parties would continue their reduction over a seven year period. The agreement went into operation on 1 January 1908 and was surprisingly successful, both in reducing Chinese production and in bringing the Indo-Chinese trade to an end. This finished earlier than expected, with the last chest of opium shipped to China from India in 1913.[165]

It was the good progress on this front which led to Foreign Office opposition to the initial American proposals to call an international meeting in Shanghai in 1909. The civil servants saw no need for further action, given that the Indo-Chinese trade was drawing to a close. They also disliked proposals for collective action in areas where the liberal tradition of British foreign policy decreed an individual, bilateral response. They believed that American motives were more self-interested, and less purely moral, owing much to considerations of trade and strategic advantage, than the American government cared to admit. Sir Beilby Alston, a senior civil servant in the Foreign Office, was moved at one stage to minute, 'It is a pity we cannot administer opium in strong doses to the United States government, when they get on the opium war path.'[166] That was indeed the case. America had not been averse to profiting from the opium trade in the nineteenth century. From 1858 to the 1880s American nationals had been free to trade in opium in and around China. They did this as freely, although not as extensively as the British.[167] By the early twentieth century, different national motives prevailed. The USA had inherited its own colonial opium problem when it took over the Philippines at the end of the Spanish–American War; the previous Spanish rulers had used a government sanctioned scheme for the distribution of smoking opium. But this offended US missionary and temperance sensibilities and a policy of suppression except for medical purposes was introduced. In relations with China, the USA aimed to protect American trading, development, and investment opportunities by every means possible; opium suppression fitted well into that approach and was supported also by US temperance interests.

The Shanghai meeting won support in Britain from Sir Edward Grey at the Foreign Office and from John Morley, secretary of state for India and a convinced anti-opiumist. They prevailed over the reluctance of the civil servants, and so a British delegation went to Shanghai. The Commission, chaired by Bishop Brent, and with the abrasive tropical medicine specialist Dr Hamilton Wright leading the US delegation, dealt mainly with the Far Eastern situation. But several significant developments ensured that its focus was more than a regional one. One was the complexity of the opium issue. There was an increase in smuggling alkaloids of opium, primarily morphine, into China; England was the world's major manufacturing country of that alkaloid. Article 5 of the final protocol, the result of a compromise resolution agreed between Britain and America, opened the door for wider forms of control. It declared that 'The unrestricted manufacture, sale and distribution of morphine' (not cocaine at this stage) was a 'grave danger' and urged that 'drastic measures ... be taken by each government in its own territories and possessions to control the manufacture, sale and distribution of this drug'. The Americans also began to discuss how to formalize the distinction they saw between 'legitimate' medical use and 'illegitimate' non-medical use. Legitimate use was defined in terms of Western medicine and science, with a lack of cultural sensibility. The colonial powers recognized the reality of alternative forms of use, such as smoking opium, and objected to such moves.

The Shanghai Protocol of 1909 had no binding force, but the Americans devoted all their energies afterwards to widening its compass and producing a treaty which would be enforceable. In September 1909 the State Department contacted governments which had attended Shanghai expressing interest in convening an international conference to lead to an international drug control treaty. The response from many countries was less than enthusiastic. In Britain, Sir Beilby Alston opposed what he called 'another gathering of opium wiseacres'. Domestic politics precluded an outright refusal, so Britain adopted some clever delaying tactics, insisting that the regulation of morphine and cocaine be more fully discussed than it had been at the initial meeting. This was partly a diversionary move intended to hamstring the American plan and to divert attention away from opium use in the Far East and in India. But it also arose out of genuine concern in both the India and Colonial Offices about the growth in morphine and cocaine smuggling in the Far East. In July 1910 for example, the Colonial Office drew the attention of the Foreign Office to the growth of morphine and cocaine smuggling in the Straits Settlements.[168] The topic was then taken up by the Americans as an important part of the international control agenda. When the US reply accepting this addition came back in September 1910, Alston commented wryly, 'It is amusing to see how our criticisms and conditions on which we have accepted the invitation have been adopted as the reasons for the conference being summoned by the USA'.[169] The conference met in 1911 and a convention was agreed in 1912, The Hague Opium Convention.

The decision at The Hague that opium, morphine, and cocaine and their use should be confined to 'legitimate medical purposes' was a crucial one for future international control. This was a significantly different stance to the defence of both medical and non-medical use, and the difficulties of distinguishing one from the other, adopted in 1895 by the Royal Commission on Opium. Also of future significance was the refusal of the German government, in alliance with its cocaine industry, to adhere to a convention which might be partially applied and therefore detrimental to her manufacturing interests.[170] She insisted that the convention had to be ratified by all thirty-four participating powers, however small and insignificant, whether they had pharmaceutical industries or not, before it could come into force. The Hague Convention assumed an 'all or nothing' complexion which the British delegates, who included Sir William Collins, the anti-opiumist doctor, Liberal MP, and later president of the Society for the Study of Inebriety, recognized in their report.

> The Shanghai Commission directed itself mainly to the subject of the opium traffic in the Far East, and was primarily concerned with rendering assistance to the opium suppression movement which the Chinese

Government had lately initiated. The present convention goes far beyond this. It has dealt with morphine, cocaine etc as well as with opium; and in prescribing measures for confining the use of the two first mentioned drugs, and others referred to in Chapter III, to legitimate medical purposes...It has, for the first time, laid down as a principle of international morality that the various countries concerned cannot stand alone in these measures.[171]

By itself The Hague Convention was only significant for those countries already committed to more stringent systems of control. The USA was at the head of those countries. It ratified the treaty in 1913 and there were moves, led by Hamilton Wright, to enact national legislation. The Harrison Narcotics Act of 1914 began Federal involvement in drug control, and was instituted as a revenue measure. Wholesalers, retailers, and doctors had to apply for a tax stamp in order to dispense drugs. But the main aim was to restrict access to drugs and to 'stamp out' addiction. Those who dispensed large amounts of drugs could be criminalized and prosecuted for maintaining addicts indefinitely, a practice which the USA wanted to end. The Act underwent numerous challenges but provided the basis on which US style prohibitionist drug control was based for decades. The Americans always cited international obligations as the backdrop to this policy.[172]

Other countries were less keen on radical change, and by the outbreak of war in 1914 there were only eight ratifications and twenty-four promises to adhere to the convention. In Britain, discussions which took place about drug control before the war and how to put it into operation did not go that far. They envisaged little more than an expansion of the existing system of regulation by pharmacists and perhaps more control of prescriptions by doctors. Many doctors did not favour greater state action—their eugenic viewpoint and belief in heredity put stress instead on building up a 'good stock' which would be resistant to drug habits. The discussion which did take place before the war was almost entirely predicated on the professional interests of doctors and pharmacists, as focused on in Chapter 4. Decisions made after discussions which took place in 1914 planned to curtail the sale of opium-based patent medicines, long an aim for both professions. Doctors were given a proviso for prescription only for the opiates and cocaine, together with limitation on the currency of prescriptions, the number of times they could be dispensed, and the total quantity of drugs to be dispensed. But this was outlined in a way which still gave pharmacists plenty of professional control. The restrictions were only to apply to a range of preparations well above the limits set at The Hague. Only medicines containing over 1 per cent morphine, heroin, and cocaine would need a doctor's prescription; under that cut off point, it would be up to the pharmacist to decide if the drugs were being bought for 'legitimate medical purposes'. Both professions remained in control, with accommodations which gave doctors more of a role than they had had before. The lead government department was thought likely to be the Privy Council Office, which had been responsible for the administration of the Pharmacy Acts, a department which had shown no great enthusiasm for further extensive legislation.

The impact of the war, however, changed all that. In Britain, it brought the justice ministry, the Home Office, into the central departmental role, and brought harsher restriction on the agenda, with a great deal of press and public concern about drug use. Two issues predominated. Smuggling increased in Europe and the Far East; and, at home, the spread of recreational use, in particular among soldiers, caused concern. Smuggling of drugs was not just a wartime matter but it became a more serious concern during the war, and also demonstrated how national controls were indeed interdependent at the international level. One country's lack of control made ripples across the international pond. Britain was still the major manufacturer of morphine, and the exported drug was diverted into China via Japan. The enormous increase in British morphine exports during the war was sufficient proof of what was going on. The Home Office, which secured control of the drug control policy arena during the war, introduced a system of import/export certification designed to ensure that all drug shipments in and out of Britain had a legitimate destination. These later provided the basis of controls introduced in other countries and the systems introduced under international drug control.[173]

Morphine was the main drug being smuggled but cocaine use also started to come onto the agenda during the war. Here the efficiency of the army was the issue, for soldiers on leave in the West End of London were buying cocaine from prostitutes and other dealers. The scare first arose with Canadian troops billeted in Folkestone. In February 1916, Horace Kingsley, former soldier and convict, and Rose Edwards, a London prostitute, were given six months' hard labour for selling cocaine to Canadian soldiers there. The Army brought in an emergency control order but soon the cocaine issue popped up again in London. Police-informer information pointed to 'ten boys who sell cocaine to the girls' working the area round Shaftesbury Avenue, Charing Cross Road, and Leicester Square in the centre of London. A case brought under the Pharmacy Act against the frontman in the network, a former porter at the Cafe de Paris, was dismissed, despite ample evidence of his cocaine dealing. Police and army pressure was accompanied by an intense press campaign which added new dimensions to the fear of 'the other'. The *Daily Chronicle* wrote of soldiers crawling into chemists' shops to obtain the drug.

> It is driving hundreds of women mad. What is worse, it will drive, unless the traffic in it is checked, hundreds of soldiers mad.[174]

The result was a regulation passed under the Defence of the Realm Act in 1916, regulation 40B, which tightened domestic controls beyond those envisaged pre-war, with a particular focus on cocaine. Germany, Canada, and other countries instituted similar controls during the war. Subsequent enquiries in Britain did not substantiate the need for such restriction. Nine months after the regulation came into force there had only been a minute number of prosecutions; a committee which looked at the prevalence of the habit as part of an enquiry into the use of cocaine in dentistry came to the conclusion that

> We are unanimously of the opinion that there is no evidence of any kind to show that there is any serious, or, perhaps, even noticeable prevalence

of the cocaine habit amongst the civilian or military population of Great Britain. There have been a certain number of cases amongst the oversee (sic) troops quartered in, or passing through, the United Kingdom, but there is hardly any trace of the practice having spread to British troops, and, apart from a small number of broken down medical men, there is only very slight evidence of its existence among the general population.[175]

But the ad hoc arrangement introduced in 1916 continued after the war and took on a permanent life of its own. Article 295 of the peace settlement enacted through the Treaty of Versailles in 1919 brought The Hague Convention into operation and gave the newly established League of Nations general supervision over international narcotics agreements. At the first League assembly an Advisory Committee on Traffic in Opium and other Dangerous Drugs was created; its original European members were France, Britain, the Netherlands, and Portugal (China, India, Japan, and Siam were the others), countries with opium monopolies in the Far Eastern colonies. It was this international agreement which, at a stroke, swept away all the pre-war difficulties about ratification and brought worldwide control. Opium and cocaine were part of a process which often happens at such times of crisis. War, and fears about the sapping of the strength of the military machine, can open the door more swiftly to actions, to regulation or legislation, which might otherwise be contentious, take much longer to put into operation, or indeed, never be passed at all. This was a crucial moment for those drugs, which emphasized and accelerated their divergence from the other substances.

How that divergence would work in practice was of course still dependent on events and on particular national factors. The convention even when put into force actually required relatively little and the colonial powers were still in control. But it did fundamentally alter the rules of the game both internationally and in terms of different national situations. Let us look at what happened nationally first. Countries which wanted to extend control and to introduce a prohibitory approach could do so, using its requirements as justification. This is what happened in the United States, where decisions under the Harrison Act in the 1920s were justified by reference to international obligations. In Britain the result was compromise: a hybrid medico-penal system emerged. The control of drugs was the responsibility of the Home Office, which had also managed the inebriates acts pre-war. Attempts by the newly established Ministry of Health (1919) to exert control were brushed aside and the task, in the view of Sir Malcolm Delevingne, Under Secretary in the Home Office responsible for drugs, was simply 'stamping out addiction' in the way the Americans were doing it.

Delevingne wanted an authoritative statement that the prescription of drugs to addicts was not legitimate medical practice. But to obtain this, he had to turn to the medical profession and to the central state agency, the Ministry of Health, to arbitrate on what was indeed legitimate. Doctors in the UK had established greater leverage with the state than in the US system. In Britain, his initiatives led to the establishment in 1924 of the Departmental Committee on Morphine and Heroin Addiction as a Ministry of Health committee. This move brought the Ministry into an important mediating role. It might not have been the lead department, but it was a major link to doctors in practice and its Regional Medical Officers had already been involved in dealing with cases of doctor addicts. It was a medical civil servant in the Ministry, Dr E. W. Adams, who was secretary to the committee, drafted its report, and set the tenor of the response. Adams was concerned to protect disease views of addiction and a doctor's professional status. Thus he wrote:

> If the addict is unwilling to enter into the relationship of patient to physician, but admits that he is merely coming to obtain supplies of a drug which he cannot otherwise get, then it is the clear duty of the doctor to refuse the case. But if the habitué desires treatment as a sick person for the relief of his pathological condition, the physician must be allowed to use his discretion.[176]

Adams' views were supported by leading members of the committee. Its chair was Sir Humphrey Rolleston, president of the Royal College of

Physicians and an exponent of disease views. Another member, Professor W. E. Dixon, Reader in Pharmacology at Cambridge, had written forcibly in *The Times* in opposition to attempts to foist the American model of drug control on British doctors. A dissenting voice to their views came from Sir William Willcox, adviser to the Home Office, and a group of prison medical officers. Their addict clientele was distinctively different from the middle class, often medically connected, patients seen by the other members of the committee. The end result was an official statement that the long-term prescription of drugs to addicts for the purposes of treating their addiction was legitimate medical practice, a statement of principle often referred to as the 'British system' of drug control. The name of Rolleston is still revered in the more liberal wing of the drug arena today; the International Harm Reduction Association in the early twenty-first century still awards the annual Rolleston Memorial Prize.

In reality, the Report symbolized an alliance between medical profession and state, but with the Home Office as well as the Ministry of Health. One commentator called this a 'system of masterly inactivity in the face of a non-existent problem'.[177] Medical expertise was established but within a framework of criminal justice. Doctors kept control of their patients who, in turn, accepted their definition of expertise. If the problem—of who was perceived to be addicted—had been different, then the solution might well have been as well. Such compliant middle-class addicts aroused little of the fear which had been evoked by opium smoking. As we will see in the following chapter there were addicts who aroused fears in the 1920s and 1930s: their existence underpinned the criminal justice side of the British policy response. As we will see in Chapter 8, the profile of addiction in the United States seems to have been different by the time of the First World War, with a decline in compliant middle-class addicts and the rise of an ethnic lower-class subculture, which also helped to determine a harsher policy attitude.

At the international level, the postwar settlement marked significant developments. The pharmaceutical industries in participant countries such as Britain, France, and Japan had expanded during the war in order to fill the gap left by lack of drug supplies from Germany. Those industries began a period of growth and also of influence at national and international levels which paralleled the process we have seen with alcohol interests in the pre-war years. International control did not stop smuggling although it did bring to an end the embarrassment it had caused to British manufacturers of morphine. Smuggling between nation states continued, with Japan as a major player in the 1920s and 1930s, again allied to imperial interests. As Japan expanded into Korea and then to Manchuria, it discovered the pull of the drug trade. Japanese subjects had been smuggling opium into China in the 1890s, but as Japan expanded its territories there, the trade assumed new importance. The big corporations and also the Imperial government itself smuggled not just opium but also the alkaloids, first morphine and then heroin. During its Asia-Pacific War (1931–45) the trade grew in importance. Profits from smuggling funded undercover operations against Chinese territories outside Japanese control, but were used primarily to finance Japanese client states in occupied China. The Japanese used opium because it raised money—as it did also for others including Chinese war lords, criminals, the Guomindang (the Nationalist Party), and even the Chinese Communist Party.[178] The interwar years saw a change in the way in which the illicit trade operated. During and just after the war, it depended on the diversion of legally manufactured drugs. By the end of the 1930s, professional criminals had taken over the beginning of the process, owning clandestine drug factories around the world.[179] Control focused on the control of the drugs supply, making it inevitable that the profits of trade would be increased, that illicit trade interests would move in, and that political interests of various sorts, either anti- or pro-government forces, or governments themselves, would move in to fill the gap as previously established participants moved out. The interwar period saw the beginnings of regular involvement by such interests in the clandestine trade.

International control also had another knock on effect. It established a mechanism which, almost by accident, brought other drugs within its ambit. In the 1920s, cannabis was the first example of this. The drug, although widely used in the East, did not figure much in European medicine in part because of the lack of identification of an active principle. It had been mentioned in discussions prior to The Hague Convention but did not form part of the final agreement. At the second Opium conference which gathered in 1924, the Egyptian delegate, Dr Mohamed El Guindy, forced cannabis on to the agenda. He did this despite opposition from the British, by aligning himself with the United States, a powerful ally, who, although not a member of the League of Nations, exerted considerable influence in a 'consultative capacity'.[180] El Guindy's sudden interest in the matter in the 1920s was a direct outgrowth of a British report on hashish smuggling and the use of the drug in Egypt. The British government had not been at all keen to make the report public because of its potential for embarrassment; for Egypt had been directly governed by Britain until 1922. El Guindy seized on the information for exactly that reason, also using statistics produced from the Cairo lunatic asylum, where it was said 41 per cent of all confined cases were caused by the use of hashish. Dr Warnock, Director of the Cairo asylum for nearly thirty years, from the mid 1890s, had produced statistics shortly after his arrival identifying what he called 'hasheesh insanity' as a major problem among the inmates of the asylum. Warnock also made sweeping assertions about the implications for the whole country—'The use of cannabis indica in Egypt seems to have graver mental and social results than in India and is responsible for a large amount of insanity and crime in this country.' James Mills has drawn attention to the generally suspect nature of the Warnock data—'his method of establishing that an individual at his hospital was a cannabis user was suspect and the conclusions that he drew about cannabis use in general were based simply on the small sample of all of Egypt's many users that had ended up in his hospital.'[181] Nonetheless cannabis controls were part of the International Opium Convention of 1925.

Between 1919 and 1925, international drug control became what William McAllister calls a 'going concern'.[182] A whole new regulatory machinery was created in the interwar years. Between 1924 and 1931 several drug treaties were drawn up. New control bodies were created. In 1929 the

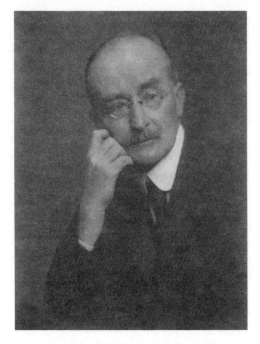

FIGURE 6 Sir Malcolm Delevingne.

Permanent Central Opium Board began its work; it was composed of eight experts, appointed in their personal capacities, not as government representatives. They included Sir Malcolm Delevingne, the acerbic British civil servant from the Home Office who had been instrumental in securing the lead policy position of that department in the UK. His influence on the international scene over a lengthy period from before the 1914–18 war and into the 1930s was profound. The international drug control machinery became a 'gentlemen's club' of men like him, of national and international civil servants. However, the chair of the Board, Herbert May, was an American and stayed in contact with the US State Department. The United States remained a powerful player, but on the outside of the overall system because of its failure to join the League. The colonial powers with their monopolies and European countries with expanding pharmaceutical industries dominated the drug control machinery in the interwar years. The USA was dissatisfied with the League control machinery which seemed to be dominated by the very colonial powers whose opium interests it had sought to undermine. It withdrew from the 1924 Geneva conference, but nevertheless its tenacity ensured that its approach began to dominate in the 1930s. Three fundamental tenets underpinned the US stance: that use other than for scientific and medical purposes was a moral and social evil; that the only legitimate transactions were those designed to meet those needs; and finally, that the basic solution was in restricting the production of raw materials to the quantities necessary to meet the world's legitimate requirements. The US approach defined a way of approaching international control which persists into the present. In particular its focus on supply and the producer countries rather than demand in countries such as the USA has attracted long-lasting criticism.[183] Such beliefs operate in the present with attempts at crop substitution in Afghanistan, as they did in the 1960s when the CIA was involved in the opium trade during the Vietnam war.[184] In Chapter 11 we will look at how international control has developed since the Second World War.

So internationalism and war, and the interlocking aspects of the role of opium in the Far East, as a national, regional, and a global substance; alongside industry interests, fear, and moral concern all combined in this period to accelerate the removal of opiates and cocaine from mainstream culture, or even from medical culture in countries such as the USA. What happened to alcohol? Did it also come under an international control regime? Of all the substances, at first sight this would seem to be the substance most poised for extensive control. To some degree that did happen at the national level in particular countries, the USA most obviously with its policy of prohibition in the 1920s. What was different was the way our two key factors in this chapter—internationalism and war—operated. Their interaction brought a rather different outcome for alcohol.

Alcohol control was also a matter of international concern before the war, as opium had been. The equivalent to the Shanghai Opium Commission was the regional control arrangement focused on Africa arrived at in the General Brussels Act of 1889–90. The main concern of that Act was dealing with the slave trade and alcohol was an ancillary provision.[185] The regulations prohibited the import and manufacture of distilled liquor. Not all areas had prohibition; in some, economic control was exerted through import and excise duties. Exceptions were also made for the non-native population since it was thought that it was not alcohol itself but African characteristics which accounted for the dangerous effects of drinking. This was in contrast to the opium debates where a universal vision of what constituted 'medical' use began to be applied to all nations. The participating nations had to report to an office in Brussels. Revisions of the agreement in terms of increases on duty were adopted at conferences held in 1899, 1906, and 1912. An International Temperance Bureau was also established in Lausanne in 1909 (the forerunner of the later International Council on Alcohol and Addictions or ICAA) to coordinate the alcohol efforts and R. Hercod, its Director, was a prominent advocate of international control for alcohol.

After the war the system fell under the League of Nations as part of its responsibility for the administration of the former German colonies. Under a system of covenants, other nations became responsible for former German territories in Africa and also responsible for the liquor traffic. This was confirmed by a postwar Convention on the Liquor Traffic in Africa which was adopted at St Germain en Laye in September 1919 and which replaced the earlier Brussels Act. The US, Belgium, Britain, France, Italy, Japan, and Portugal signed the convention and there was some tightening of controls, in part because of the illicit traffic which the earlier agreement had given rise to. The League of Nations had oversight of the mandates through a Permanent Mandates Commission composed of experts, not considered government representatives, from the signatory countries.

The similarities with the Shanghai/Hague process are obvious—but also the differences. The scheme remained a regional one, despite calls in the 1920s for it to be expanded into a system like international drug control. R. Hercod speaking at the international conference against alcoholism in Geneva in 1925, said

> When the League of Nations was founded, one question of necessity arose in the fighters against alcoholism: could not and would not the new international organization, which does not confine itself to political aims but displays a beneficent activity in the fields of public hygiene and philanthropy, interest itself in the alcohol question? ... Are not alcohol and opium both narcotic drugs and cannot their effects be compared? If the League of Nations does such splendid work against opium why would it not do the same against alcohol?[186]

The difference was obvious by this stage. International control for alcohol remained an African based regional system which never made the transfer to a global system. What was lacking—by comparison with the opiates and cocaine—were several key components—industrial interests pushing for a global system, cultural concern or fear, amplified by war, and timing. The Hague Convention of 1912 had put in place an incipient global system for drugs before the war; no such event occurred for alcohol.

War did have a clear impact but this was at a national level, and was not allied, except in a limited way, to an emergent international system. Again, as with the opiates and cocaine, there were clear differences between British and American forms of national control. In Britain, wartime concern about the effects of drink on the war effort and the changing position of working-class women in the labour market brought not prohibition, but central state regulation.[187] Whether drinking was indeed hampering the war effort to quite the extent it was said to be is a question which has been debated by historians. But the issue was adroitly used by Lloyd George, then minister of munitions, who at one stage considered state purchase of the whole liquor trade, a strategy which in part grew out of the pre-war moves bringing temperance and the trade together through the idea of moderate reform and 'disinterested management' which had been on the agenda before the war, as we saw in Chapter 3. Drink nationalization proved not to be practical politics; instead a Central Control Board (CCB) was set up in 1915. Separate from the 'vested interests' of trade and temperance, it was given wide powers to regulate or even purchase the trade in key military and naval areas. It limited the hours of consumption and introduced the famous 'afternoon gap', when pubs and clubs had to close. 'Off' sales of spirits were prohibited in the evenings and at weekends and a policy of dilution of the strength of spirits was introduced. 'Treating' in pubs was prohibited to deal with the problem of servicemen being plied with excessive numbers of drinks. A research committee was set up and the Board, chaired by Lord D'Abernon, was concerned to base its initiatives on scientific evidence. It began to expand its remit to seek a more general solution to intemperance and the problem of the licensing system. State control of the trade was introduced in certain areas such as Enfield in north London and the Cromarty Firth and Gretna area. The war thus saw the local introduction of a system of 'disinterested management' within a framework of state control. As John Greenaway has commented, 'The work of the CCB showed what could be achieved when positive policies towards alcohol were undertaken by a government department.'[188] Statistics showed that such policies, widely accepted by the public, had a major impact on measures of harm from alcohol such as deaths from cirrhosis of the liver and arrests for drunkenness.[189] Trends apparent since the 1890s were accelerated.

Like drug control, the CCB was a temporary wartime expedient. Unlike drug control, it did not continue and expand postwar. Some of the elements of the wartime system remained in existence through a licensing Act passed in 1921, but central control was abandoned. Divisions between different interest groups prevented a continuation of the wartime system. In the United States, in contrast, the national situation was different and war led to a system of prohibition which continued after the war. Nationwide prohibition began in 1920 following the passing of the 18th Amendment to the American Constitution and its subsequent enactment in the Volstead Act. US prohibition has had a bad press; it came to an end largely because of the Great Depression which took hold from 1929. The prospect of substantial revenue from taxing alcohol, during a time when the taxable economy had shrunk, was hard for the government to resist. Industrial and business interests, who had originally thought that prohibition would deal with injuries and absenteeism, also no longer supported prohibition as they had once done. But its results were not all bad; the often used mantra of 'we all know that prohibition didn't work' needs qualification. In areas such as the rural South and West, where there was support for the laws, they were effectively enforced. Overall, Americans drank less and alcohol related disease fell. There were other prohibition related changes. Spirit drinking expanded (spirits were easier to transport than beer), women's drinking expanded as part of more general trends, and the old style saloon with its heavy drinking culture came to an end. On the negative side, organized crime and political corruption flourished and deaths from poisonous illicit alcohol use increased. The law divided the older Protestant order of rural interests, focused on temperance and abstinence, from new immigrants, Italian or Irish Catholics, arriving as part of rapid industrialization and urban growth in the 1880s and 1890s. Drink continued to be available in different forms—medicinal, illegal beer, smuggled spirits, industrial alcohol, and production from illicit stills. Even so, in the early 1920s consumption had dropped to about 30 per cent of pre-prohibition levels. By the end of the decade, although drinking had increased, it was still only two thirds that of the pre-war levels.[190]

It would be wrong to say prohibition did not work. In some respects its results were beneficial. But it did show the difficulty of trying to introduce severe restriction without public support and also support from key economic interests. Repeal resulted from the onset of the Great Depression which altered voters' priorities, rather than from the characteristics of the prohibition system itself.[191] Prohibition in the USA was the best known of efforts by a number of countries to introduce similar systems. Before the war, Iceland and Finland had introduced prohibition; Canada and Norway had partial prohibition. Russia instituted prohibition during the war and Sweden voted in favour but never actually brought it into practice. The Scandinavian countries and Poland actually drew together as a bloc in the mid 1920s and called for an international convention. Meanwhile, the US had to negotiate bilaterally with countries to allow it to search vessels which it suspected of smuggling. Further attempts to take controls through the League of Nations came up against strong opposition from the French government representing the interests of the wine industry.

There was what Schrad has called a 'global prohibition wave' drawing on pre-war international temperance networks and catalysed by the war during this period.[192] In the 1920s there were attempts by US prohibitionists to extend the war on liquor. Tyrrell says that international conditions between 1917 and 1919 were as propitious as they would ever be to a worldwide prohibition drive. Even the French had

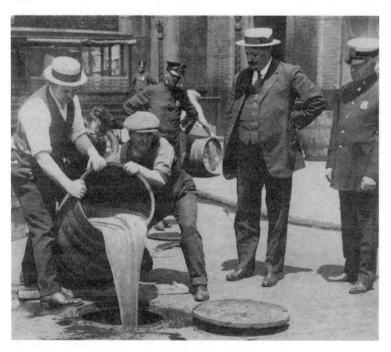

FIGURE 7 Prohibition in the USA.

banned absinthe during the war. International networks were of key importance, in particular the Womens' Christian Temperance Union (WCTU), in alliance with the World Prohibition Federation and the International Reform Bureau of Washington which had also been involved in the war against narcotics before the war. But these attempts failed because of anti-American sentiment, complex class and cultural opposition to prohibition, and negative reporting of the experiment with prohibition, in the USA.

Without the sequence of events which had brought international drug control, international action on alcohol was doomed to failure. Action on drugs at that level ultimately rested on international moral networks in combination with the economic interests of the pharmaceutical industry and of governments—and the crucial issue of timing. These factors were present for alcohol but not in the same combinations or at the same time. The absence of any clear international treaty before the war (which could then have been inserted into the peace settlement) was also crucial. And of course tobacco did not figure at all in these international control arenas, although it was the subject of wartime national controls in the UK. International control for tobacco came at the end of the twentieth century and in the early years of the twenty-first, as we will see in Chapter 11. It then emerged within a rather different framework which in turn started to impact on ideas about international drug control. But for drugs and for alcohol it was during the First World War that the combined impetus of internationalism and war conditions led to distinctively different postwar paths.

8
Mass Culture and Subculture

In a letter written in May 1915, J. W. Spearman, a soldier, explained why he smoked.

> In the trenches we smoke the whole time, except the few hours we snatch for a snooze and during the time we stand to, just before dusk and dawn. I never relished a smoke so much as when in the trenches; it keeps my mind off the snipers and controls my language when the bullets whiz by.[193]

Eighteen years earlier a female correspondent in the *Evening News* had written of what smoking meant to her.

> What can be more enjoyable than to be comfortably ensconced in a big armchair in a pretty cosy room, with a very few friends around you, discussing everything between heaven and earth while you puff your cigarette airily, lazily, dreamily, energetically, just as the theme discussed provokes you?
> How easily the thoughts come, how well one talks, how confident one feels, while following the blue clouds floating upwards.[194]

But young women's drug use was quite another matter. Here is the *Daily Express* in 1918.

> You will find the woman dope fiend in Chelsea, in Mayfair, and Maida Vale. An obscure traffic is pursued in certain doubtful teashops. The sale of certain beauty specifics is only a mask for the illicit traffic in certain drugs.

A young and attractive girl deeply interested in social conditions and political economy made the acquaintance of another woman through a mutual friend. Within three months she had become a confirmed haunter of a certain notorious cafe. She had lost her looks and health. Before she closed her miserable existence a bare nine months later she had introduced at least four other decent girls to her practice of vice; and for the last two months of her existence she was acting as a decoy for a notorious gambling hell...

The queer, bizarre, rather brilliant bachelor girl is a frequent victim to the insidious advances of the female dope fiend.[195]

Smoking opium, too, evoked a frisson. Drugs like opium, drinking alcohol, and smoking a pipe had all been culturally acceptable in some form in the middle of the nineteenth century, as we saw in Chapter 2. The issues outlined in the intervening chapters had served to push the substances down different regulatory routes. Cultural change was also entwined in that process. Culture itself is not an independent variable. Cultural changes reinforced forms of regulation, which in turn impacted on culture and helped along further changes. This chapter will look at how one substance—tobacco—became a mass cultural phenomenon in the interwar years, the 1920s and 1930s. Drugs in contrast, began to develop the beginnings of a subculture—consumption in opposition to the perceived norms of society, in a way which deliberately challenged or tried to subvert those norms. In the interwar years it is perhaps premature to speak of a fully formed drug subculture, but nevertheless, the implications of drug taking were very different to those of smoking, which began a period of mass cultural acceptability. This chapter does not deal with alcohol, which both in Britain and in the USA, was less important in the interwar years. In the USA that decline in consumption may have been connected with prohibition, but in Britain, its declining use can be connected in part with wartime controls but also a change in social and leisure habits.

We left tobacco-smoking culture back in the mid nineteenth century when men smoked mostly pipes and cigars, women used clay pipes or snuff, and cigarettes were still hand rolled. Industrialization and new technology made mass-produced cigarettes more easily available and numbers smoking them rose in the first half of the twentieth century. As we have seen, there was no international control mechanism for tobacco as there was for drugs. Consumption rose among both women and men, but smoking was overwhelmingly a male habit. In 1920 the annual consumption of cigarettes per woman was too low to record, and it compared with a 44-a-week average consumed for each man over fifteen. Women's smoking rose rapidly to 180 a head annually by 1930 and 500 by 1939, so that it can be estimated that all women of fifteen and over were smoking nine cigarettes a week. On the eve of the Second World War, women were smoking nearly forty times as many cigarettes as in 1921, although this was still only 14 per cent of male consumption.[197] Cigarette smoking had become a mass cultural phenomenon by the time the war was over. By 1949, there were estimated to be 21 million cigarette smokers in Britain, 13.5 million men and 7.5 million women. Of every 100 men in 1949, 81 were smokers and 39 out of every 100 women.[198]

Smoking was overwhelmingly a male activity at this stage, although women have borne the brunt of attention in discussions of these years. In the First World War *The People* newspaper called on its readers to send Woodbines—'Tommy's favourite fag'—in bulk at prices as low as ten for a penny, or else contribute to their massively subscribed 'Tobacco Fund'. In 1937 the survey organization, Mass Observation, conducted research in what they called 'Worktown' (actually Bolton in Lancashire) and, with an anthropologist's eye, examined every aspect of everyday life. They scrutinized smoking habits because these were part of working-class life, and even produced a book called *Man and His Cigarette*. Main cigarette smoking occasions were after meals, at social events, before breakfast, and as a stimulant. Cigarettes were an aid to social interaction and this was a central function, seen again and again. One smoker had persisted with the habit for eight years in order to be part of the group, although in fact he had never enjoyed smoking. He kept cigarettes in stock in order to offer to friends to give an air of liberality.[199] Such attitudes persisted in the postwar period in the most unlikely places. Sir Austin Bradford Hill, the pioneer smoking researcher, was still accustomed, even after the publication of the path-breaking research in the 1950s, to keep a box of cigarettes to offer to visitors in his room at the London School of Hygiene and Tropical Medicine. When the health service researcher Walter Holland asked him why he did this, given the harmful effects of tobacco that his own research had demonstrated, Bradford Hill's reply was 'But it would be impolite not to offer a cigarette.'[200] Smoking was embedded in a set of cultural rituals which have been relatively little studied. Smoking a cigarette was seen as manly, and about attaining adulthood and taking one's place in the adult world; smoking was a public display of masculinity. Boys would be given a symbolic pack of cigarettes by their fathers when they reached the age of transition to adulthood—somewhere between fourteen and sixteen, dependent on working lives. George V gave his sons cigarettes at sixteen and he had smoked in his teens.

Cigarettes were at the centre of elaborate male rituals. In the pub, for example, the offering of cigarettes to friends helped to define the group: 'It enclosed a community to the exclusion of non-smokers and continued that public, communal mode of consumption associated with pre-industrial cultures but which survived through and beyond the nineteenth century.'[202] But smoking cigarettes was a cross-class activity, as was pipe smoking, although with these differences.

Pipe smoking became a cross-class activity during the 1920s and 1930s but it was the cigarette which became the emblem of mass culture. In a rare set of oral history interviews done with elderly smokers in Glasgow, smoking was overwhelmingly seen as a masculine habit. This informant was recalling the 1930s and 1940s.

> When they all came out of the Clydebank shipyard, all these men, with their wee bunnets on, they all had cigarettes. The wives didn't have money for the cigarettes. The wives had to keep the children, but the men always seemed to get their cigarettes.[201]

Certain brands became associated with certain types of smokers. The major part of interwar cigarette consumption was in the middle-priced brands—6d for ten. Players became the mass brand par excellence with

Players Medium a mass cigarette. From just before the war until 1943, it was claimed that every second smoker bought Players. Players built a new factory in Nottingham in the 1930s employing 7,500 people. The Players sailor image was ubiquitous. However, they were not quite as popular in the north of England, where Woodbines were the favoured cigarettes of industrial workers. At 4d for ten, these appealed to people on low incomes.

The rise of mass advertising and other forms of marketing paralleled and underpinned this mass culture. Although initially reluctant, British tobacco companies joined in the overall expansion of consumer advertising from the late nineteenth century. Tobacco advertising rose noticeably in the 1920s and 1930s with well-known brands from WD and HO Wills (Woodbine, Goldflake, and Capstan), Player's (Navy Cut), Gallagher (Park Drive), and Carreras (Black Cat). £30 million a year was spent on advertising in the 1920s, rising to a to peak of £60 million in 1937. New promotion strategies by the companies from the late 1920s were key to this. By the 1930s cigarettes were available from branches of Woolworths and other department stores. Film shows promoted cigarettes; planes with trailers in the sky advertised them and neon signs emblazoned cigarette brands. Packaging and embossed cartons replaced the newspaper in which the handrolled cigarettes had been wrapped. Coupon cigarettes were a major marketing technique. Reintroduced by Carreras in 1925 they accounted for one-third of all cigarette sales by the time they were banned in 1933. There were cigarette cards and children's painting books given away with cigarettes. The coupon was a particularly successful technique, giving, as Penny Tinkler has put it, cigarettes a useful role in the domestic economy, and promoting them even among people who did not smoke. One advertisement for Carreras Black Cat cigarettes featured a woman showing off the non-laddering stockings her boyfriend's or husband's coupons had obtained,

> Molly told me about them first; I admired a pair she was wearing and couldn't believe her when she said she got them for coupons from Black

Cat cigarettes. So I asked Dick to smoke 'Black Cats' (the silly boy was always changing his cigarettes) so as to get me a pair. He just grumbled—but he tried 'Black Cats', and now he swears by them and will smoke nothing else. I'm perfectly satisfied too.[203]

Advertising tapped into the interwar fashion for health and fitness—the health-giving properties of tobacco were widely advertised.

Women smoking was part of this expansion of consumer culture but the actual role of smoking among women in the 1920s and 1930s should not be overestimated. Smoking had been expanding among both working and middle-class women since the 1880s. The First World War, with the greater independence it gave to women, also speeded up this trend. Smoking spread among munitions workers and nurses. There were specially produced 'ladies cigarettes' some with gold-tipped mouthpieces, and scented with violets and roses. Factory girls smoked 'brownies' sold at three for a halfpenny. Older forms of smoking also continued—the use of clay pipes and of snuff. Older women in Preston, Barrow, and Lancaster interviewed by Elizabeth Roberts for her oral histories used snuff. However, women largely smoked the same brands as men.

Outside, visible smoking by women was becoming more common and images of women smoking began to appear in advertisements by the end of the 1920s. Women smoking in the cinema was well established by the 1930s and heroines were flourishing cigarettes. The glamorous women in films all smoked—Mae West, Marlene Dietrich, and Tallulah Bankhead. But women smokers were nowhere near as widespread as men. Smoking was still a defiant type of activity for a woman. One girl started smoking at dances in the 1920s 'for effect and to appear grown up—i.e. at dances where in those days in our circle parents were present and some of the elderly women would look rather disapprovingly at girls who smoked.'[204]

Smoking was associated with rituals as it was among men. But these were different. Lipstick left on a cigarette stub was seen as vulgar. Men would light women's cigarettes; they did not light their own. Smoking in the street was definitely not respectable for women.

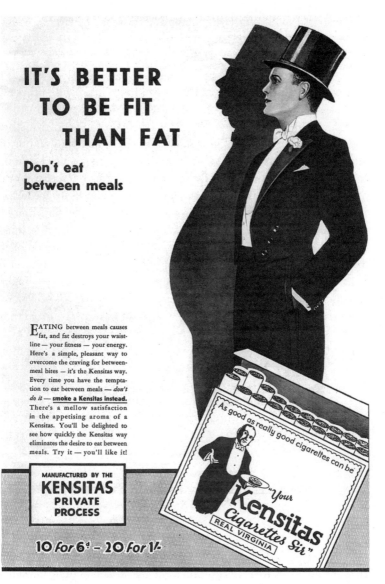

FIGURE 8 Tobacco advertising in the interwar years.

Alice, one oral history respondent, started smoking in her late teens in the 1940s and 1950s

ALICE: You didn't smoke in the street, ladies, women didn't do that, you didn't smoke in the street, you'd have to be sitting down maybe having a coffee or after your meal, you know an occasional one.
INTERVIEWER: Do you know why that was?
ALICE: It just wasn't sort of lady like, it just wasn't accepted, just the same as women didn't go into pubs in those days.[205]

It was during and after the Second World War that the big expansion in women's smoking took place. Despite a number of government measures to reduce civilian consumption and protect supplies to the troops consumption nevertheless rose by 20 per cent among men and 150 per cent among women by the end of war. The decades from the 1950s to the 1970s was the time when smoking among women was most acceptable and at its highest level.

In an early anti-smoking book, *Common Sense about Smoking*, published as a paperback in 1963, the politician Lena Jeger gave a good sense of what smoking meant to young people and to girls.

Smoking provided

something to do with their hands...some little social grace of contact, the ice-breaking which comes with the offer of a cigarette. The pause in conversation can be covered by the striking of a match, the stubbing out of a cigarette end, the filling or knocking-out of a pipe. If people have nothing to say to each other, silence seems less awkward if they are smoking. Friendliness is suggested by the closeness of two heads bent over a light. Social confidence makes these things matter less, but they cannot be underestimated...

As far as girls are concerned, there have of course been times when it was considered a gesture of 'progressive defiance', a touch of bohemian daring. The pity for girls is, however, that smoking is about the most stale and unattractive way of asserting that one is uninhibited, emancipated, or even fast. Smoking was always a pretty poor symbol of modernity, for Indian squaws have smoked through the centuries.[206]

How far the mass advertising and marketing strategies of the tobacco companies caused this expansion of consumption among both men and women has been much debated. Were they creating demand and duping consumers? One American historian of smoking, Allan Brandt, has written of what he calls 'the engineering of consent' among women by the advertising and public relations strategies of the tobacco industry in the interwar years.[207] Advertisers had realized the potentially vast extent of the female market by the 1920s. In 1928 American Tobacco spent $7 million to advertise its brand Lucky Strikes. Here was a prime example, so he argues, of the 'creation of needs'.

> Smoking for women…became part and parcel of the good life as conceived by the American consumer culture and explicitly represented in advertising campaigns.[208]

Here was the 'artificial creation of desire for the purposes of profit'. A public relations agency employed by the tobacco companies, Bernays and Hill, tried to alter norms around smoking, for example, in relation to smoking in the open air or on the street. Nor was this limited to Hill and American Tobacco—by the early 1930s the major US tobacco companies had all enlisted professional marketing experts and were spending large sums on advertising. Philip Morris cigarettes were popular after their introduction in 1933 for this reason. It was through this branding and mass advertising, so Brandt argues, that cigarettes became a part of mass culture in the USA, especially among women.

This type of argument is powerful and has been much used also by public health advocates in their later campaigns for the restriction and banning of advertising. It argues for the 'duping' of consumers, and tends to see them as the passive recipients of advertising messages. This was also a view put forward by theorists of mass culture in the Frankfurt School of the 1920s and 1930s who believed in the power of the mass media to indoctrinate its recipients in the population.

But this line of argument is rather one-sided. One criticism of the approach is that the 'voice of the consumer' is absent. We do not hear what smoking cigarettes meant to consumers in the ways in which Mass Observation and oral history interviews tell us in the UK. There are other differences between the UK and the USA too. Commentators have cautioned, using newer theories of the 'impact' the media has, about overestimating its power and also that of the mass advertising it contained. Newspapers expanded their circulations in the interwar years and there were battles for readership. Display advertising became a feature of the press, which became more dependent on advertising revenue. The main part of advertising in the British papers, aside from the 26 per cent spent on financial and real estate, was directed at the domestic consumer. The media historian Adrian Bingham notes the increased prominence of female bodies used as sales techniques—this period saw the sexualization of women in many of the outlets of mass culture. But he concludes 'It is important not to exaggerate the coercive effects of advertising'; the coercive power of the press has been over-estimated by commentators and historians.[209]

Penny Tinkler, who has studied women's smoking and its representation in the media, comes to similar conclusions. Smoking was a growing habit among women before they started to be targeted. There is no evidence of intentional targeting of women among British companies before the mid 1920s. But Tinkler recognizes the possible influence of advertisements not targeted at women—for these could have shaped their views and aspirations. Authors like Tinkler argue that the effect of advertising cannot be isolated and its effects measured. But it certainly contributed to a culture where tobacco use was 'normalized'. One Mass Observation informant, Brenda Pool, stated—'I didn't take a liking to the actual tobacco for some time—just to the act of smoking.' The language and practice of smoking was established as common parlance with a new importance for the visual and visual cues.[210]

Mass advertising and promotion of brand images contributed to the expansion of the smoking market in the interwar years and thereafter. But they were not the only cause. Those who assess the impact of mass health education campaigns in the present day argue that they can be effective in promoting behaviour change, but only if they build on issues already inherent in culture and develop areas of pending cultural change. In the case of cigarette smoking, we also need to isolate factors such as the impact of both world wars on men and women, a new companionability and sociability built on greater freedom and equality for women and more leisure time for both sexes. Readers of newspapers and viewers of advertisements made sense of them in a complex way—incorporating them and decoding them according to their own values and norms. It is unwise simply to talk of 'indoctrination' by the mass media, or by the tactics of the tobacco industry—that would be far too simple an analysis of a complex series of interactions.

There was no such mass culture of drug use in the interwar years, despite the visual allure and portrayal of the allied practice of opium smoking. In a country like China, where opium use had been ubiquitous, a rapid process of decline set in, later accelerated by stringent government action after the Second World War. In Britain, there were no mass advertising campaigns, brand promotion, or public relations discussions. Instead we can see the elaboration of what became, after the Second World War, a fully fledged drug subculture. Before that, three phases can be identified: recreational drug use in literary circles in the decadent movement of the 1890s; the extension to broader circles during the First World War; and then the drug scene of the 1920s and 1930s. Even then there was hardly a group (with one or two exceptions) with a way of life centred on drug use. Drugs were still mostly an incidental part of wider literary upper-class and artistic interests—aping French literary fashion in the 1890s or the vogue for the USA in the 1920s.

As cigarette smoking was emergent as a mass activity in the 1890s, some forms of drug use were becoming part of the 'new aesthetics', which rested on a denial of society, a retreat into the individual with an emphasis on separation and inner consciousness and experience, in contrast to the vulgar materialism of the external world. The aesthetic movement brought with it an increased interest in the occult and paranormal, and thus in drug use. The Society of Psychical Research (1882), the Theosophical Society, the Fellowship of the New Life (1884), the Rosicrucian Society of England, a small group of master Masons with a penchant for the occult, were all part of a trend which encompassed changing consciousness and also changing society. The Rhymers Club was the literary wing of the decadent movement, and was one of the main vehicles, together with the mystic groups, through which recreational drug use was promoted.

Cannabis and opium, both of which were smoked, were the main drugs used at this stage. It is interesting to reflect on the different cultural milieu within which 'smoking' was positioned at this stage. Smoking cigarettes, at least for 'new women' also had some counter cultural elements. W. B. Yeats, one of the founders of the Rhymers Club, took hashish while in Paris in the 1890s, and other members of the Club also took the drug, including the writer Ernest Dowson. During an afternoon tea party given by the writer Arthur Symons in his London rooms in Fountain Court, Dowson, the writer John Addington Symonds, and some of Symons' lady friends from the ballet, all tried hashish. Symonds, who at this period was earnestly pursuing 'experience' in all its variety, with love affairs, visits to low pubs, the music hall, and foreign travel, described the event.

> On the following afternoon, Dowson turned up, then the ballet girls one after another, whose laughter and whose youth always enchanted me; then Symons, whose entrance seemed to disturb them, then began to be curiously nervous and by being for a few minutes nervously shy. Yet when, with the gravity of a Doge, he handed round the tea, and I the cakes and cigarettes, we suddenly became quite at home. Later on we tried the effect of hashish—that slow intoxication, that elaborate experiment in visionary sensations, which to Dowson at Oxford had been his favourite form of intoxication, which, however had no effect on him, as he sat, a little anxiously, with, as his habit was, his chin on his breast, awaiting the magic, half shy in the midst of that bright company of young people, of which I was the host and the gatherer, whom we had seen only across the footlights.[211]

The use of the drug was a self-conscious literary aping of French fashions. The hashish use in France of writers and artists such as Gautier, Charles Baudelaire, Gerard de Nerval, Rimbaud, and Paul Verlaine stimulated similar trials in England.

The circles were small. Arthur Symons' rooms in Fountain Court was the location for drug use of various sorts including opium smoking about which he wrote in the poem, 'The opium smoker'.

I am engulfed, and drown deliciously.
Soft music like a perfume, and sweet light
Golden with audible odours exquisite,
Swathe me with cerements for eternity.
Time is no more. I pause and yet I flee.
A million ages wrap me round with night.
I drain a million ages of delight.
I hold the future in my memory.[212]

Symons also had a temporary lodger in the 1890s, Henry Havelock Ellis, a pioneer social scientist and theorist of homosexuality who was interested in the relationships between dreams, visions, and drugs. The drug mescal appeared to have the ability to evoke a dream-like procession of visual imagery and in 1896, Ellis began to experiment with it in his lodgings in the Temple. Yeats, who was lodging with Symons at the time, and Dowson also took part in the trials. Ellis published an article on the experimentation 'Mescal: a new artificial paradise' which appeared in the *Contemporary Review* in 1896. He retained an interest in the drug and published further on it in the early 1900s. His interest predated that of Aldous Huxley in LSD (the active principle of mescal), described in *The Doors of Perception* in the 1950s.

One feature of this experimentation with mescal and also of the use of hashish and opium smoking was that the boundaries between 'orthodox' medical and 'unorthodox' recreational or non-medical use were still difficult to define in the 1890s. Literary experimentation was akin to medical experimentation; several of the protagonists had medical backgrounds and there was a long tradition in medicine of self-experimentation to test out drugs. Ellis himself had been a medical student at St Thomas' and his mescal use had been prompted by studies published in the medical journals. Dr Weir Mitchell's 'Remarks on the effects of Anhelonium Lewinii (the mescal button)' read before the American Neurological Society in 1896, had been reprinted in England.[213] Weir wrote that after taking mescal:

The display which for an enchanted two hours followed was such as I find hopeless to describe in language which shall convey to others the beauty and splendour of what I saw.

To take it was an 'unusual privilege' and he saw the drug as useful for the emergent science of psychology—a view which led to further experimentation later, in the 1950s.

By the First World War, this limited recreational use had expanded. Drug users now included theatrical and artistic circles with connections to upper-class Bohemians, and with military connections during the war. To hashish and opium smoking were joined cocaine as the new recreational drug of the period. In 1901 the deaths of Edith and Ida Yeoland, two unemployed actresses, who died from overdoses of cocaine, had given an indication that recreational use might be spreading among a broader artistic clientele. The wartime drug scare in London outlined in Chapter 11 had further shown the extent of the West End street trade. These drug using circles came more clearly into focus in the Billie Carleton case of 1918–19, which was mentioned in Chapter 5. In the Carleton circle, opium smoking parties and cocaine sniffing were all the fashion. Billie herself, Reggie De Veulle, Lionel Belcher, a 'cinema actor', and his girlfriend, Olive Richardson, were a group of artistic film and theatre people who, in Richardson's words, experimented with drugs 'absolutely for the fun of the thing'. There were connections with army officers on leave and passing through London. Jack May, American proprietor of Murray's Club in Beak Street, was organizer of West End dances for officers and was said to have introduced Billie to opium smoking.

The drug culture had expanded to include theatre people, army officers, aristocrats and artists. It remained upper class. Cocktails, parties, meetings at the Coq d'Argent in Soho, drug dealing at the Café Royal in Regent Street, and visits to Limehouse were all part of the extended postwar scene. The 'drug novels' of the period give a flavour of the climate, among them Sax Rohmer's *Dope: A Story of Chinatown and the Drug Traffic* (1919), Lady Dorothy Mills' *The Laughter of Fools* (1920), and G. P. Robinson's *Testament: The Confessions of a Drug Taker* (1922). *Dope* was loosely modelled on the Carleton case. The tale involved Monte Irvin, a city alderman and prospective a marriage proposal to Rita turned down, and had introduced her to drugs—cocaine, veronal, and opium smoking. Chandu (opium) smoking parties were held in the Duke Street flat of Cyrus Kilfane, an American comedian appearing in London. One such party was officiated over by Mrs Sin, or Lola, the wife of a Limehouse Chinese modelled on Mrs Ping You in the Carleton case. Rita's drug habits led her into other byways—visits to Limehouse for drug dealing with Sir Lucian and to a doctor no longer recognized professionally but recommended by a lady friend addicted to the use of the hypodermic. A mysterious Home Office investigator intervened, empowered to enquire into the drug traffic by the Home Secretary, Lord Wrexborough. His pseudonym was '719' but he turned out to be Seton Pasha, formerly a Foreign Office person and a 'sound man to have beside one in a tight place'. Matters moved to a thrilling denouement. Pasha and Inspector Kerry, an upright policeman, traced a drug warehouse in the East End and cracked the syndicate which had gained control of the market. Mrs Sin killed Sir Lucian (they had had an affair previously in Buenos Aires); she in turn was strangled by her husband with his pigtail.

The story was melodramatic but corresponded with the picture which emerged from other sources. Augustus John, the painter, frequented the Café Royal in Regent Street, which seems to have been a drug taking milieu, and spoke of drug taking parties in Hampstead with Iris Tree the actress and her husband Curtis Moffatt, where hashish was consumed in the form of a compote, along with sardines and wine.

The Freda Kempton case in 1922 also evoked memories of the Carleton affair and brought the drug scene to public attention again. The death of this young nightclub dancer led to an inquest where it was revealed that she had taken cocaine and phials of the drug were found in her flat. There was also Chinese involvement again—not Limehouse seamen, but the far more dapper person of 'Bill' or 'Brilliant' Chang, owner of a restaurant in Regent Street and with connexions in the West End smart set. It was Chang who was alleged to have supplied Freda with cocaine. The case was followed by the conviction in 1923 of Edgar Manning, a black drug dealer, and brought anti-alien feeling to a height.

There was considerable police pressure against cocaine dealing in the West End. Chang was sentenced for possession of cocaine and deported in 1924 and a new Dangerous Drugs Amendment Act in 1923 brought a harsher line for drugs offences.

Cocaine was the recreational drug of the period. The bisexual Duke of Kent took cocaine during an affair with Noel Coward in 1920s.[214] Nicky Lancaster, Coward's cocaine taking character in his play *The Vortex* premiered in the 1920s, symbolized the hectic and nervy pace of postwar upper-middle-class life. The popular press amplified the role of drugs in this emergent culture. The *Daily Express* in 1922 was typical. The signs of drug taking could not be easily erased.

> They cannot alter the expression of the unfortunate deluded habitués living in their pitiable paradise of sensation. They cannot cast clothing over the immodesty of the half clothed young girls, they cannot make the drug fiend and his associates look like clean men.[215]

The British Board of Film Censors and the London County Council (LCC) banned a film called *Cocaine* which was based on the Kempton case. The film showed, again according to the *Daily Express*, 'sleek young men and thinly clothed girls…[who] jazz and shimmy and foxtrot under the influence of late hours and excitement, nigger-music and cocktails, drugs and the devil'.[216]

We can get an idea of which groups were using drugs in a way which came to the attention of the police. In these years the British government started reporting on drug prosecutions to the new League of Nations Opium Advisory Committee. In the 1920s, there were three distinct groups of users—cocaine users, opium smokers, and those using morphine. It was really only cocaine which showed a pattern of subcultural use. Those prosecuted for cocaine offences in the 1920s indicate that the trade was a street one centred on the West End of London, as illustrated by the case of Britannia Yettram, who was prosecuted for selling cocaine in 1922.

> Police sergeant Marks stated that the prisoners were seated on a Thursday evening in the lounge of the Shaftesbury Tavern, a public house on

Shaftesbury Avenue, and together four women approached Yettram and went upstairs with her, remaining a few minutes and then leaving the premises. The first-comer said to Yettram, 'Got it?' while another enquired 'Any snow, Gipsy?' and Yettram, who is also known by the name 'Gipsy', replied that she had.[217]

There was no 'Mr Big' with perhaps the exception of Chang for a while and the cocaine itself seems to have come from a variety of sources—some diverted from legitimate possession by doctors or dentists, some smuggled in from Germany and Merck. It came into the country in 'numerous trickles rather than a single torrent'.[218] Often it was associated with key figures. Jack May, for example, of Murray's club in London, continued his nightclub and drug supply career in the interwar years in a new Murray's club in Maidenhead, where cocaine could be obtained.[219]

The other major 'illicit' group, although of course there was overlap on the West End scene, were those prosecuted for smoking opium. Opium cases provided the majority of prosecutions (57 per cent) in the 1920s and over 80 per cent of those cases were in London, Liverpool, and Cardiff, with their connections to trade in the Far East. Most of the offenders were male, many were seamen or laundry men and in the prosecution tables they almost always had Chinese names. These Chinese were prosecuted for possession or for smoking opium, with the punishment more usually being a fine or deportation rather than prison. In July 1922, the police raided an opium den in Limehouse and prosecuted the proprietor, Low Ping You, whose wife, now dead, had been involved in the Billie Carleton circle four years before. He was recommended for deportation. The testimony of Mr Cecil and of Annie Lai, both quoted in Chapter 5, tells us about the opium-smoking scene from the 1900s to the 1920s.

With the exception of the West End 'set' who visited Limehouse this was far from a drug subculture. Nor was the third group of those prosecuted (likely to be under-represented in the statistics because of the UK's primarily medical response), who were those taking regular doses of morphine. These cases were older than the others—an average age in their forties, and a quarter were female. These cases occurred outside

London and were more geographically scattered; over 60 per cent were medically connected: doctors, chemists, or nurses. But a quarter were technical offences—professionals failing to keep records in the way in which the Acts required. The other set of offences involved individual addicts trying to obtain a drug from a chemist through forged prescriptions. Behind these statistics lay a different type of drug consumer, who had been catered for by the provisions of the Rolleston Report in 1926, as outlined in Chapter 7. These were respectable, professional addicts who had been addicted therapeutically and wanted to remain within that milieu. Thomas Henderson, the son of a well-known Edwardian artist had been addicted to morphine for nearly forty years and called at the Home Office himself in 1922 to put the case for continued prescription.

> I claim to be a useful life to the state, teaching others to earn their living and only asking to be permitted to earn my own, and I appeal to you…to see with unbiased eyes, and I implore you…not to crush me out under this new law…Morphia has not corrupted me…it has never tempted me to do wrong in any respect…I only ask to be left in the hands of my doctor.[221]

This was the group of addicts who accepted the professional authority of their doctor and who were very far from a subculture.

One exception was Lady Diana Cooper (formerly Manners), a friend of Iris Tree, who seems to have used morphine for the fun of it. Diana had 'doped' with chloroform—'jolly old chlorers' and also with morphine. She and Katherine Asquith took the drug together. Diana told Raymond Asquith in 1915 that her only moment of pleasure in the previous month had arisen when she and Katherine had lain

> in ecstatic stillness through too short a night, drugged in very deed by my hand with morphia. O the grave difficulty of the actual injection, the sterilizing in the dark and silence and the conflict of my hand and wish when it came to piercing our flesh. It was a grand night, and strange to feel so utterly self sufficient.[222]

Diana's fiancée and later husband, the politician Duff Cooper, noted in his diaries that they had quarrelled because of her wish for morphine which he had refused. The ostensible reason, in July 1919, was that she had broken her leg. He recorded 'the chief trouble...is to cure Diana of taking morphine. She has been having it ever since her accident and now cannot do without it. Every evening there is a scene until she gets it.'[223] However, it seems likely her morphine taking had a longer history and for less than therapeutic purposes.

Illicit drug use in Britain was on the wane after the strenuous police activity of the 1920s against cocaine and smoking opium. Morphine-using 'therapeutic' addicts continued their careers largely out of the public eye. So was there any subcultural use at all? Some commentators have seen nothing until post Second World War, with the growth of the more familiar drug scene of the 1960s. But there were some addicts whose lifestyle centred on drug use. Aleister Crowley was one. Crowley had been involved in the magical circles of the 1890s. He was a friend of Allan Bennett, a chemist later turned Buddhist monk, who introduced Crowley to the potential of mind-expanding drugs and the recreational use of cocaine. His strident defence of recreational use continued into the 1920s. A poem 'Morphia' (1914) and a piece published on cocaine in 1917 were followed by two articles published in *The English Review* in 1922 and *The Diary of a Drug Fiend* published in the same year. Crowley's articles were 'The great drug delusion' by 'A New York specialist' and 'The drug panic' by 'A London physician', the latter supposedly a response to the first article, although in fact both had been written by Crowley himself. He argued that repressive legislation would only lead to increased production of drugs and police corruption. Crowley opposed the belief that addiction was inevitable. He tended to ovestate the opposition case.

> I attempted to produce a 'drug habit' in myself. My wife literally nagged about it: 'Don't go out without your cocaine, sweetheart!' or 'Did you remember to take your heroin before lunch, big boy?' I reached the stage where one takes a sniff of cocaine every five minutes or so all day long; but although I obtained definitely toxic results, I was always able to abandon the drug without a pang.[224]

In his *Diary*, he provided an accurate picture of the 1920s scene with thinly disguised portraits of Augustus John, Iris Tree, the sculptor Jacob Epstein, the writer Frank Harris, Lord Alfred Douglas, and others who frequented the 'Café Wisteria' (or Café Royal). With chapters on 'A heroin heroine' and 'Au Pays de cocaine' Crowley attacked drug control and the general regulation of postwar society. The language of drug use—'snow', 'H', 'cold turkey'—underlined the creation of a separate drug using argot and identity. Crowley cut a rather ludicrous figure as he continued his belief in 'Do what thou wilt shall be the whole of the law' and stoked his media-inspired reputation as the 'wickedest man in Britain' throughout the interwar years. But he did represent a new type of figure—the exclusive addict.

Nor was he an isolated figure. Despite the tailing off of cocaine and opium smoking prosecutions in the 1920s, there were networks of addicts whose life centred on drugs and how to obtain them. One such was the circle centred on Brenda Dean Paul, the daughter of a baronet and a Polish pianist, whose Bohemian career as an addict extended into the 1950s. Dean Paul had been a neighbour of Noel Coward's in Ebury Street in London in the 1920s and her subsequent career took in involvement in literary and artistic circles including association with the fashion designer Cecil Beaton and the actress Hermione Baddeley, whose partner, David Tennant, became Brenda's lover. Her visits to Berlin and Paris in the 1920s and 30s brought with it an introduction to cocaine, morphine, and heroin, and also many run-ins with the law back in Britain. Dean Paul became a 'drug celebrity' actively collaborating in the construction of her own exclusive addict identity through the media. A Sunday paper financed her ghosted memoirs, which were published in 1935 as *My First Life*. Publicity photos for the book showed a ravaged face, sunken eyes, lined cheeks, and skeletally thin limbs. She visited the USA in order to lecture the young on the evils of drugs, which she continued to take. In the 1930s the artist Michael Wishart saw her in the Kings Road in Chelsea 'with her silver mane and slacks, scarlet mouth and man's overcoat to match, tottering with her friend Miss Baird to refill her hypodermic syringe'. In 1950 at his wedding party held at the artist Francis Bacon's studio in Kensington, she danced in high silver heels, scarlet trouser suit, and dark glasses. Brenda 'wilted habitually at the approach of midnight when she and her friend Jean would disappear…to return…with a simple white powder, which they dispensed generously with a thimble to our wearier guests'.[225] The image was emblematic of later 'heroin chic'.

So the British picture so far as drugs were concerned was a group of iatrogenic (medically induced) addicts most often using morphine, and very small 'junkie' networks, exemplifying lives focused on drug use— together with some recreational use of a wider range of drugs in literary and artistic circles. In America the culture was different, even before the First World War. The very different form of government regulation in the USA and the different stance of American doctors underpinned and helped to shape a different form of drug using culture. The American historian David Courtwright has argued that medical and therapeutic addicts were a dying breed in the early twentieth century in the States, even before the Harrison Act, as doctors grew wary of prescribing opiates and cocaine and as newer drugs came on the market. What he calls the 'more disreputable types of users', notably opium smokers and sniffers of heroin, came to predominate. By 1940, the dominant type of addict was a young lower-class male, using heroin or morphine and the majority of cases were non-medical.[226] Doctors were reluctant to prescribe opiates, and this tendency was intensified by the 1914 Harrison Act. The number of non-medical addicts increased in proportion to medical ones. Heroin in eastern cities and morphine or morphine with cocaine was used elsewhere in these circles. Two doctors in Chicago looking back over more than 5,000 cases they had treated between 1904 and 1924 remarked,

> Fifteen or twenty years ago, most addicts acquired the habit through physical disease or discomfort. Today the number of new addictions through physicians' prescriptions is small. The great majority of cases now result from association with other addicts, following their advice in taking a 'shot' or a 'sniff' for 'what ails you' and searching for new sensations. These are the pleasure users.[227]

The descent down the social scale also had an ethnic dimension. Heroin use became widespread in the immigrant slums in the 1910s and 1920s. Mel, the only child of poor black parents, born in 1915, gave an idea of the New York drug scene in the 1930s.

> I started dealing in 1934. I was selling heroin, coke, morphine. I had a bankroll. I found a guy that handled it by quantity, so I just went and bought some. I bought me an ounce or two. I'd make three, four hundred dollars a week. That's one way I'd support my opium habit.
>
> I was selling from Thirtieth Street to Thirty-fifth street, about five blocks on the West Side. I sold from my apartment–you know, telephones and things like that....
>
> When I first started dealing I had Chinese and Jewish connections: later I had Italian connections. It was a beautiful thing when the Chinese and the Jews had it. But when the Italians had it—bah!—they messed it all up.[228]

The lower-class ethnic subculture was entirely different to the scene in Britain, where the tiny group of Chinese opium smokers provided the only ethnic dimension. This was a key difference between Britain and the United States during much of the twentieth century.

The interaction between regulation, the role of the state in drug control, and the underlying culture of use is a complex one. Drug use had started to descend the social scale in the USA and to become a lower-class criminally related activity in the early years of the twentieth century. Subsequent professional disengagement with the area, regulation, and international control intensified those trends. So regulation did not create culture in a simple way. The wider context was a very different type of society, with great waves of immigration and also a strong Protestant prohibitionist ethic. All of this was absent in the UK; general practitioners remained involved and the morphine using professional addict remained more prominent into the postwar years. Subcultures differed between these countries. But the broad contrast between mass smoking culture and subcultural opposition to dominant culture for drugs was common to both. Drugs had become detached from mainstream culture.

9

The New Public Health

The divergent cultures for tobacco and for drugs which developed in the first decades of the twentieth century, and in the 1920s and 1930s in particular, brought to an end the significant period of regulatory and cultural repositioning which had begun in the mid nineteenth century. By the interwar years of the twentieth century, professional interests, economic and technological change, fear of users, social movements, and international regulation—or lack of it—had sent the substances down divergent paths. Tobacco had become an item of mass culture, while the response to drugs had been repositioned within a medico-criminal justice framework, in the context of international drug control. The impact of the First World War had provided a significant impetus to new ways of looking at the substances, drugs in particular. The culture of alcohol consumption remained a mass one but not at the level experienced in the nineteenth century. Levels of consumption in the UK began to fall significantly from the last quarter of the nineteenth century and remained low until the 1960s.[229] Despite a rise in living standards, people chose not to spend their new income on drink and new leisure pursuits became more popular.

The frameworks established during and after the First World War were not immutable and began to change again after the Second World War. The final chapters of the book (Chapters 10–12) will examine another period of repositioning then. The 1939–45 war was less

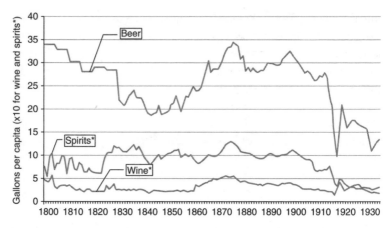

FIGURE 9 Alcohol consumption in the nineteenth and twentieth centuries.

significant for the substances than the First World War had been. For drugs on the international scene, however, it did bring the United States much more centrally into drug control through the postwar international control machinery. US support for the Mafia in Sicily and Marseilles as an anti-communist force enabled the organization to establish a significant base in the postwar heroin trade. John Collins' research has shown how it was US pressure which led the colonial powers to abandon their opium monopolies after the war and to fall in line with a prohibitionist approach towards international control.[230]

New forces after the war also impacted on tobacco and its cultural use, which is the focus of this chapter. Tobacco began a process of detachment from mainstream culture which accelerated from the 1970s. Tobacco began to develop the same sorts of associations over time as illicit drugs; what had been a mass culture of tobacco smoking began to look more like a subculture on the drugs model. Tobacco became a 'loser's drug'. This chapter examines how some of the factors identified for alcohol and illicit drugs also came into play to begin the marginalization of tobacco after 1945. The role of science and professional groups, activist movements, fear, and internationalism all came into the picture. The more recent accommodation of tobacco and illicit drugs and the pending involvement of alcohol is a process we will look at in the concluding chapters.

The key to the repositioning was the change which took place in public health after 1945. This chapter will look at how tobacco became a public health issue in those postwar years and how that substance came to epitomize new directions in public health. Tobacco's marginalization came through science, but down the professional route of public health epidemiology, not through medicine and the disease theories applied in the late nineteenth century to drugs and alcohol. The factors identified in previous chapters began to impact on tobacco from the 1950s and helped to begin the process of detaching it from mainstream culture.

Science and professional interests were in this case those clustered around the new version of public health. The scientific and professional backdrop was the change in public health after the war. Whereas for alcohol and for drugs in the nineteenth century, pharmacists and doctors had been the professionals involved, for tobacco a century later, the driving force for change came from public health personnel and the new public health speciality of chronic disease epidemiology. Changes in the nature and definition of public health stimulated the change. For what was termed 'public health' had not stayed the same over time. In the eighteenth century, public health initiatives had begun on a local basis, with attempts by city governments to deal with environmental problems, such as ensuring fresh water supplies, air quality, and the removal of waste. These efforts intensified in the nineteenth century, when rapid economic growth and mass urbanization coincided with high mortality from infectious diseases such as cholera and typhus. The role of the central state emerged, with a body of law and administrative practice which focused on managing and modifying the environment to lessen the risk of disease. Public health at this stage was an environmentally focused affair, using sanitation, the provision of drains and water closets, as a key tactic, and it was more the realm of engineers than of doctors. As we have seen in previous chapters, drugs and alcohol had only a small part to play in nineteenth-century public health. There was concern from public health interests about the 'doping' of children with opiates and the connection between this and women's factory work. Some of the early medical supporters of the disease-focused Society for the Study of Inebriety were public health doctors, Medical Officers of Health, including the Society's president, Norman Kerr. But drugs and alcohol were never mainstream public health issues at this time. The overwhelming importance of temperance as a social movement against alcohol meant that there was relatively little discussion of that substance specifically as a public health issue. Tobacco had hardly figured in public health discussion at all.

The environmental emphasis in public health had declined in the early twentieth century. The scientific breakthroughs of the 1860s, when the French chemist Louis Pasteur had formulated germ theory, had opened up other possibilities for investigating disease in a more specific way. The broad environmental emphasis gave way to one focused more on the individual in the home—and that individual was most often the mother, responsible for the wellbeing of the family and the 'future of the race', in the eugenic terminology of the time. Health education of individuals rather than improvement of the overall environment, became a key public health tactic in the early twentieth century. Throughout the interwar years, when public health doctors in the UK were running health services in a proto-national health service, public health academics had debated the wider role of public health. The doctrine of social medicine, important in many countries in the interwar years, envisaged a broad role for a reformulated public health, which would ensure that the promotion of health would underpin the provision of health services. Such hopes were dashed in the UK, where public health as a profession did not take over the management of the new health service as exponents of social medicine had hoped.

Patterns of disease were changing in the postwar world. Deaths from infectious diseases were declining and the old killer diseases such as tuberculosis were disappearing. Mortality from cancer and heart diseases assumed a greater prominence. Public health underwent a further period of reorientation and redefinition around this new era of chronic disease. The dilemmas and the new approach were expressed in this extract from a radio talk in 1955 by Jerry Morris, one of the pioneers, both of social medicine and also of the new style of public health.

> We are dealing with a different social situation. The nineteenth-century epidemics, bred in poverty and malnutrition, arose from the failures of the social system...But coronary thrombosis...with its origins apparently in high living standards...seems to be arising from what we regard as successes of the social system...It is becoming clear that in the modification of personal behaviour, of diet, smoking, physical exercise and the rest, which look like providing at any rate part of the answer, the responsibility of the individual for his own health will be far greater than formerly. It will not be possible to impose from without (as drains were built) the new norms of behaviour better serving the needs of middle and old age. They will only come about in a new kind of partnership between community and individual.[231]

The focus of public health was becoming what individuals could do to avoid the onset of 'self' as opposed to environmentally induced disease. The technical key to the new postwar public health was a revised style of epidemiology, the traditional public health tool of the study of disease in populations. The new epidemiology dealt with chronic rather than infectious disease and began to use a new terminology of 'risk' and the 'risk factor'. Rather than direct causation of disease, the immediate impact of germs as agents of infection, public health personnel began to concentrate on the role of long-term risk factors that might bring about ill health in the distant future rather than immediately. The importance of what became called 'lifestyle', that is, individual behaviour and habits, began to be stressed and how these could be modified. Initially governments found the transition in their relationship with citizens—from preventing infectious disease to advising on changes in personal habits—a difficult one.

Smoking and its connection with lung cancer provided the initial case study for this new approach to public health and opened up the new era of 'risk' and lifestyle. Smoking emerged as a key health issue in the 1950s and 1960s in both Britain and the United States. Of course, health problems connected with smoking had been discussed in the medical journals pre-war—smoker's heart for example. In Nazi Germany, health promotion initiatives had included action against tobacco based on research and the American biometrician Raymond Pearl had also studied the connection in work undertaken for the insurance industry. Postwar, two sets of researchers, Wynder and Graham in the USA, and Sir Austin Bradford Hill and Richard Doll in the UK, a statistician and an epidemiologist, were the first to demonstrate the connection. Doll himself, a radical social medicine advocate who was a member of the Socialist Medical Association and the Communist Party until the 1950s, always maintained that discovering the connection between smoking and lung cancer was a surprise.

> [W]e began our study without any expectation that tobacco was likely to be an important cause of the disease and we included questions about its use primarily because the consumption of tobacco and particularly the consumption of cigarettes had increased at a possibly appropriate interval before the increase in mortality began to be recorded. For my part, I suspected that if we could find a cause it was most likely to have something to do with motor cars and the tarring of the roads.[232, 233]

There had been a gradual increase of cancer; a change in the balance of the sexes with cancer, towards men; and increasing prominence of lung cancer as a form of cancer. The greatest increase in that cancer had come in males over forty-five where the cancer had increased six fold between 1930 and 1945. In Britain, concern about this rise was aroused in the Ministry of Health and the Medical Research Council, and had led to the funding of a research study carried out in the Statistical Research Unit of the London School of Hygiene and Tropical Medicine, the leading public health institution and a powerhouse of statistics at this time. The results, published in the *British Medical Journal* in 1950, concluded that there was a 'real association' between carcinoma of the lung and smoking, and that smoking was a factor, and an important one, in the production of carcinoma of the lung. The work was based on a case control study of twenty London hospitals and the conclusions were cautious. Later, in 1956, came the results of a prospective study of doctors which the two researchers initiated in 1951. This study related the deaths of doctors to groups which in 1951 were non-smoking, currently smoking, and ex-smokers. The study concluded that the death rate for lung cancer increased as the amount smoked increased, and that there was a reduction in mortality with the increase in the length of time over which smoking was given up. This 'doctors' study' continued to report its results over the next forty years, with results from the follow up published in 2004, just before Doll's death the following year.

Here was the new science which was eventually to lead to the marginalization of tobacco. But in the 1950s there was widespread uncertainty about what this evidence meant, in particular for politicians used to a laboratory-based style of proof. Tobacco tax was an important component of government revenue at that time, 16 per cent of central revenue in 1950. In 1954, the Minister of Health, Ian Macleod, remarked, 'We all know that the Welfare State and much else is based on tobacco smoking.'[234] Politicians were also wary of being seen to give advice to the public about a condition which might never manifest itself, or only after many years. The issue was taken forward through pressure from outside government. A key role came from health professionals both in Britain and the USA, with a report from the Royal College of Physicians, *Smoking and Health*, published in 1962 and another two years later from the US Surgeon General. The issue's focus moved from an environmental one to one focused on the individual. The British College's committee was originally set up to look at smoking and air pollution—both were thought to be implicated in the rise in lung cancer. But air pollution was left out of the committee's initial considerations and its final report, because it raised more difficult issues at that time. The science was unclear, the relationship with policy was difficult and it was likely to fall foul of the industrial interests whose polluting habits would be attacked. Domestic air pollution had just been dealt with by the 1956 Clean Air Act and so it was seen as unwise to pursue the air pollution issue further at that stage. Smoking, on the other hand, was an individual habit which could be more easily modified, or so it was thought.

The key players at that time in the anti-smoking coalition give a sense of the professional and scientific interests who opposed smoking. The lead player was the deputy Chief Medical Officer (CMO) Sir George Godber, who encouraged interests outside government to take up the issue in order to build up a head of steam which government could not ignore. The range of membership of the RCP committee underlined the heterogeneity of professional interest in the issue and the professional networks forming round the new risk-based public health. Key members were Charles Fletcher as secretary, son of Walter Morley Fletcher, former secretary of the MRC, with impeccable medical connections, but also a talent for communicating with the public through the media. That emphasis on the media was shared with another member of the committee, Jerry Morris, the social medicine advocate and public health epidemiologist, whose advocacy of media and advertising initiatives on the committee was notable. These were medical and public health modernizers with a social conscience, some of whom had been based at the Central Middlesex Hospital in London, a powerhouse of social medicine sentiment.

Here was the professional and scientific impetus which we talked about in relation to drugs and alcohol in the late nineteenth century. There the outcome had been medical agitation for an alliance with the state over treatment through the inebriates acts. For tobacco in the 1960s the agenda was very different; the RCP report's agenda was consumerist and media focused. Of seven demands, five were for public education; restrictions on sales to children; restriction of tobacco advertising; tax increases and perhaps differential taxation for less harmful pipes and cigars; also information on the packet about the tar content of cigarettes. Only two were different; restrictions on smoking in public places and the 'medical model' of anti-smoking clinics.

The manner of the report and its launch were also media oriented in a way which was unusual for the time. The RCP hired a public relations consultant to manage the launch and held its first ever press conference. Charles Fletcher later remembered the splash the launch had made.

On the day before publication a press conference was held at the College and it was crowded. Many questions were asked. When one reporter quoted that the annual risk of lung cancer in heavy smokers aged 55 was only one in 23 the president asked him if he would fly with an airline only one in 23 of whose planes crashed he agreed he would not. Next day there was fortunately no big news and the report got major headlines.[235]

This trading of the statistics of the relative risk of activities was something new in postwar discourse—but would become a commonplace in the media presentation of health issues as time went on.

Tobacco in the interwar years had epitomized the new role for the visual in public life. As science identified these risks, the agenda for government action also became a visual and media focused one. There was a ban on television advertising in the mid 1960s and later a requirement for a government health warning on packets. But the main focus was on advertising and the mass media approach. Initially there were rather old-style efforts at local health education with a van campaign in 1962–3 which disseminated anti-smoking propaganda throughout the country. But this was also the dawning era of mass persuasion, with models coming from social psychology and the use of American theories about the impact of advertising. Health education in England was reorganized in the late 1960s and a central body, the Health Education Council, was set up to manage the new mass media approach. The Council's establishment was preceded by an official government report, the report of the Cohen Committee in 1964. The report envisaged a new breed of health educator who would be part salesman, persuading people to take action on health risks. Training the public would involve both imparting knowledge and imparting self discipline—a key phrase in the new style of public health. It also involved persuading the public about the right action to take through national mass health education campaigns. In the early 1970s the Saatchi brothers, later to become a major advertising company, first made their name through advertising campaigns they ran for the Health Education Council. Those on smoking attracted particular attention. Early in 1970 Saatchi produced advertisements showing 'The tar and discharge that collect in the lungs of the average smoker'; and 'You can't scrub your lungs clean.' The *Sun* newspaper noted how dynamic and brutal the copywriting was. Advertisements in 1971 showed smokers crossing London's Waterloo Bridge interspersed with pictures of lemmings throwing themselves off a cliff. A voiceover said:

> There's a strange Arctic rodent called a lemming which every year throws itself off a cliff. It's as though it wanted to die. Every year in Britain thousands of men and women smoke cigarettes. It's as though they want to die.[236]

The Saatchis ran a campaign for the HEC about pregnancy with a doleful pregnant man fronting the strap line 'Would you be more careful if it was you that got pregnant?' The smoking counterpart which ran in 1973 was a striking image of a naked pregnant smoking mother to be fronted with the text 'Is it fair to force your baby to smoke cigarettes?' Large sums of money were spent—around two million pounds by the mid 1970s—small beer by comparison with the expenditure of the tobacco companies on advertising, but much larger sums than had been expended when health education was a local matter, paid for out of the rates. To this new direction in public health were added new styles of research and investigation—market research and social surveys which looked at the attitudes of the population or at the ways they had responded to the campaigns. A whole new industry of pre- and post-campaign testing and evaluation was coming into being, bringing survey research and psychology into the realm of the new public health approach. This was far from the treatment and disease model which had conceptualized alcohol and drug use as medical 'problems' decades before.

Other destabilizing factors also came into play. Social movements in the nineteenth century had been epitomized by the mass movement of temperance, which had helped to undermine alcohol consumption. Action against tobacco had been weak at that time, confined to the National Society of Non Smokers (NSNS) a small organization whose members tended to be dismissed as 'cranks'. Anti-tobacco in the new era of public health postwar developed a much more effective social movement. This was ASH (Action on Smoking and Health) set up in 1971 by the Royal College of Physicians after a further report on smoking, *Smoking and Health Now*, had been published. Government had wanted something like this to happen so that they could use it as a rationale for action. A leading civil servant in the Ministry of Health, Enid Russell Smith, had written in a memo in 1962:

> There is at present very little in the way of an anti-smoking lobby and it may well be that at the present intermediate stage, when the nature of the connection between smoking and lung cancer has still not been fully established, the most effective measure to limit smoking would be the promotion of a voluntary anti-smoking movement. It would be much easier for the Government and the local authorities to take regulatory measures against smoking if there were a body of opinion pressing them to do so.[237]

ASH was a very different movement to temperance. For a start, it was hardly a movement at all. It was one of the new style of voluntary organization or pressure groups of the 1960s and 1970s, part of the era of 'new social movements'. Funding came from the Department of Health rather than from grassroots supporters and the main aim was to make waves in the media rather than to hand out tracts or organize mass rallies. Its second director, Mike Daube, imported this style from his previous job at the housing charity Shelter, where he had worked with Des Wilson, doyen of the new style of campaigning. In an interview in the mid 1970s he recalled the direction he gave to ASH:

> It seemed to me when I came into ASH that here was a pressure campaign that was ripe. It hadn't been properly used. You had your villain. You had your St George and the dragon scenario, you had your growing ecology bandwagon, growing interest in consumerism. It seemed there were a lot of prospects of making something out of it.[238]

Daube made the new organization's name through media 'stunts'—buying one share in a tobacco company, then turning up at the AGM to ask about its profits, with attendant media publicity; cooperating in television programmes, *Dying for a Fag, Licensed to Kill*, or *Death in the*

West, all of which aired in the 1970s. Stirring up media storms was a stock in trade. One such was over a new low-tar cigarette called Westminster Abbey. Daube suggested to a journalist that she contact the real Abbey to see what they thought of the name: they of course knew nothing. Daube then phoned up the Abbey spokesman, who remarked that they had just had a journalist enquiring. Daube responded that this showed how wide the interest and concern about the new product was. A report appeared in the journal *Adweek* and the Dean of the Abbey sent Daube a copy. Daube complained to the Abbey, the Dean consulted lawyers, meanwhile Daube and journalists were keeping in touch. It was what he called the 'rapier and stiletto' approach—later known as 'spin'.

Like temperance, ASH was also involved in politics. It helped set up the Commons All Party Group on smoking in 1976, with members from both Labour and Conservative parties. It was what political scientists would call an 'insider/outsider' organization. Its appearance as outside pressure group was extremely useful when governments wished to claim they were under pressure on the smoking issue. In reality, connections with government were close. In the 1970s when the Labour Minister of Health David Owen was trying to pass certain initiatives under the Medicines Act, the fact that he was working closely—but secretly—with ASH, helped maintain the political momentum on smoking. In 1974, Owen had stated this plainly at a conference jointly organized by ASH and the HEC.

> The facts of life are that Government in this area will respond to pressure, and I, instead of acting defensively on the pressure that you will put me under, am coming to you with a different message, which is to say, 'Put me under as much pressure as you like.'[239]

ASH was the late twentieth-century equivalent of temperance in the nineteenth century and like temperance, or least the prohibitionist wing of that movement, it espoused a strong anti-industry stance. Daube operated, so he said, according to the American activist text, *Rules for Radicals*—'rule one is to personalize the problem—the people running the major companies are responsible for those deaths'.[240]

Part of the distinctive new public health package of measures which developed during these decades was thus hostility to industry and calls for much higher taxation of tobacco products. Here, economic factors came into play. In Chapter 6 we saw how the economic and technical developments of the second half of the nineteenth century had led to mass markets for tobacco and for alcohol, but to a more restricted market for drugs. Those mass markets were maintained, but in the UK the battleground increasingly became an economic one. The tobacco industry found it more difficult in the long term to maintain the comfortable relationship it had had with government. During the war, the British industry had been under government control and the Board of Trade had appointed Sir Alexander Maxwell, a leading leaf merchant, as Tobacco Controller. Maxwell and representatives of Imperial Tobacco, the dominant British company, worked closely with government and this relationship continued after the war. Once the results of the Doll/ Hill work were known, the objective was seen as working with government, as it had done during the war, to produce a cleaner product. To this end, research was funded via the MRC, and the industry also worked with public health researchers in what was then seen as a shared project to reduce harm from cigarette smoking. Geoffrey Todd, Imperial's lead statistician, provided information and figures for the 1962 RCP report and the report was also shown informally to the industry organization, the Tobacco Manufacturers Standing Committee, before publication.

Throughout the 1970s, industry, government, and public health researchers cooperated in a harm reduction agenda—trying to reduce or replace what was harmful in the content of cigarettes or perhaps to replace them altogether by some entirely new product—the safer cigarette. By the end of the 1970s this agenda had run into the sand. Low-tar cigarettes had been shown to be harmful as researchers drew attention to 'compensatory smoking'—smokers might be taking in more tar rather than less by smoking greater numbers of cigarettes for their nicotine content. Safer cigarettes, or products which replaced cigarettes altogether, had 'bombed' with the abortive launch of New Smoking Material (NSM) in the late 1970s.

Taxation then became a key tactic for public health activists. Initially in the 1960s and 1970s the idea had been to have differential taxation, that is, taxes which were graded according to the harmfulness of the tobacco product or the particular cigarette. But the failure to identify what was harmful and the increasing gulf separating public health and industry led to the dropping of this strategy. Public health researchers wanted higher taxes overall. The evidence on the impact of increased taxation was actually far from clear. A cross government enquiry into the impact of increased taxation which had reported in 1971 (but which was never officially published) had been presented with a Treasury memorandum which estimated an overall fall in consumption from a fivepence increase on a packet of twenty and a net loss of tobacco revenue of about £120 million. An increase in tobacco duty would increase demand as purchasing switched to other goods. It would lead to an excessive level of demand in the economy, which would have to be offset by higher taxation. The impact, it was envisaged, would fall in particular on the elderly and the poor as they would continue to smoke and would also pay higher taxation in other ways as well. The impact would also fall through higher taxation on those who did not smoke at all, affecting higher income groups most. The measure was thus likely to alienate the electorate at both ends of the income spectrum. Health figures were equally surprising—for either a 20 per cent or 40 per cent reduction in smoking the health benefits in terms of expectation of life were relatively small, but the projected effects on welfare costs were considerable.[241] There were thus political arguments in terms of electoral impact for not tangling with the taxation issue.

It was only when the electoral arguments began to diminish in the mid 1970s onward—as a decline in smoking became apparent—that taxation became a political tool. The period when Dennis Healey was Chancellor of the Exchequer between 1974 and 1979 was important in this respect. Both alcohol and tobacco came under different tax regimes. The 1974 budget introduced the notion of essential and less essential goods, with wine, spirits, and tobacco classified as less essential. The health case began to be accepted. In 1977 a voluntary agreement with the industry had them agree to drop advertising of higher tar brands and in 1978 Healey raised taxation on higher tar cigarettes, the start of differential taxation which had been long discussed. Consumption habits were affected by the higher levels of taxation and company reports thought it had led to a drop in sales. Changes in the excise tax exceeded inflation from the mid 1970s into the 1980s, added to competition from imports and unemployment. The tobacco industry began to diversify into other markets.

So the economic dimension of tobacco began to change in the 1970s. Politicians like Richard Crossman had been unwilling to introduce measures such as a ban on cigarette coupons in the late 1960s because of the unpopularity of such measures with the electorate. But in the 1970s smoking began to decline and another factor also identified as significant in the positioning of substances—fear, or connection with 'the other' began to come into play. Unlike opium smoking, racial minorities did not come into the picture, but the role of women was yet again an important one. Smoking was becoming detached from mainstream culture. Overall prevalence among adults aged sixteen and over fell steadily between the mid 1970s and the early 1980s, faster among men than among women, until there was effectively no difference between the sexes. By 1982, 38 per cent of men smoked and 33 per cent of women, down from a peak of 82 per cent for men in 1948 and a peak of 45 per cent for women in 1966. But in the 1980s the rate of decline slowed. This raised issues for industry and public health campaigners which, for both, initially focused on rights. For the tobacco industry and some pro-tobacco campaigning organizations, the issue was the rights of the smoker. After all, he or she harmed no one but themselves, or so it seemed. Smoking was a voluntary risk where smokers could make up their own minds. The public health campaigners began to fight back with a discussion of the rights of the non-smoker, a debate which began in the 1970s: ASH was collecting international information on this issue. The rights argument was, for that organization and anti-tobacco activists, a way of reintroducing consideration of the environment which smokers and non-smokers both occupied, but detaching the debate from the unwelcome 'moralizing' concerns of the earlier anti-tobacco campaigners. Organizations such as the NSNS had stressed the selfishness of smokers in inflicting their smoke on others, as for example in these lines on the tobacco habit, published by the Society.

> In how many houses all over the land
> Is tobacco the tyrant, forever at hand
> Pervading each room and polluting the air?
> So long as they're at it, the smokers don't care
> How others may suffer who cannot avoid
> The horrible fumes with which they're annoyed.
> They do not, these smokers, consider at all
> What to *them* may be sweet, may be bitter as gall
> To those who prefer to breath air clean and pure
> But who daily, and hourly, that smoke must endure.
> How *selfish* they are—what perversion of taste,
> Continuous bad manners, uncleanness and waste.[242]

Rights was a way of escaping this 'eccentric' focus on the environment. There was indeed evidence that it chimed better with public views on smoking. Local surveys and also the evidence of government social survey research on smoking underlined a high degree of support from non-smokers for the arguments that smoking in public was a nuisance and aesthetically displeasing. However, public health campaigners thought that these would carry little weight without some further form of justification which the 'value free' issue of rights seemed to provide.

Then in the 1980s, when the decline in smoking seemed to have stalled, came a new development in epidemiology and a new focus for campaigning effort. Science and the social movement came together around the issue of a new risk, that of 'passive smoking' and this re-energized the anti-tobacco movement. In 1981 papers by the Japanese epidemiologist Hirayama and others, published in the *British Medical Journal* showed that the non-smoking wives of heavy smokers had a much higher risk of lung cancer. A steady stream of publications after that date from around the world added weight to the case for passive smoking. In 1986, a US Surgeon General's report accepted the case for what it called 'involuntary smoking', and a National Academy report in the same year assessed and measured its health effects. In Britain there was an interim statement from the government's Independent Scientific Committee on Smoking and Health (ISCSH) in 1987 and in its final report in 1988 the committee accepted the case for passive smoking but with some imprecision about what effect it really had.

> [T]here might be 1 to 3 extra lung cancer cases per year per 100,000 non-smokers regularly exposed to ETS. Since there are no firm data on the number of people who fall into that category, no more than a rough estimate of the actual number of lung cancer deaths arising in this way could be made. It might however amount to several hundred out of the current annual total of about 40,000 lung cancer deaths in the United Kingdom, a small but not negligible proportion.[243]

Debate about passive smoking was intense and it was argued that the interests of the anti-tobacco movement had determined the perceived legitimacy of this scientific fact. Certainly it seemed to be a 'fact waiting to happen', science which supported the policy directions in which public health interests wished to move. Some of the leading epidemiologists in the field—Doll himself and his collaborator Richard Peto—argued that smokers should be the main concern and that passive smoking was insignificant epidemiologically. The combination of epidemiological and toxicological data underlined that public health was moving forward into new scientific areas and alliances, something which will be significant for discussion in the next chapter.

It was also a significant 'policy fact'. At a stroke, passive smoking aroused fear and expanded the notion of risk to a much wider group, potentially to anyone who came into contact with smokers. It built on gradually expanding restrictions on smoking in public. When the London Classic cinema chain had introduced these in the 1960s the restrictions were widely ignored. But the Pizza Express restaurant chain had introduced smoking restrictions successfully in the late 1970s. As Matthew Hilton has noted, the conviviality of the self-help smoking cessation group had begun to develop alongside the time-honoured conviviality of the smoke-filled pub.[244] Passive smoking as science was acceptable at a time when public attitudes and behaviours were changing; it served to reinforce these trends and to accelerate them. The climate of feeling in turn gave support to the meaning of the science. Culture and science were locked into an interactive relationship.

One reason why the science proved acceptable was that it highlighted the 'innocent victim' of tobacco smoke—either a non-smoking female married to a smoking male, or else a child or baby (or foetus earlier) who was an involuntary victim. Researchers began to connect a huge range of birth defects and failures of development later in life with the single fact of whether the child had been born to a mother who smoked or had been brought up in a smoking household. Sometimes the extent to which this was taken was quite extreme. In 1987, for example, the *British Medical Journal* published an article which purported to show differences between the appearance of babies born to women who smoked and those who did not.

> We believe that infants born to mothers who smoke can be distinguished from those born to non-smokers by their appearance. We and others could not, however, identify or quantify the difference being detected. Certainly it was not the most wrinkled or dimpled babies who were selected. Selection was by a simple subjective 'gut feeling'. Nevertheless, this finding remains useful.[245]

These approaches paralleled those in the USA where 'crack babies' were removed from their mothers, or the scientific discussion round the new area of Foetal Alcohol Syndrome (FAS) where there was similar discussion of facial appearance. Researchers seemed to be using the passive smoking issue to align tobacco use with these other substances too, something we will return to in Chapter 10.

The focus on the role of infants and children, 'the future of the race' as it would have been termed at the turn of the twentieth century, meant that the woman's role soon moved from 'innocent victim' to culpable vector of infection—the traditional role which has been outlined in the earlier discussion of alcohol in Chapter 3. The most high profile victim of passive smoking was male—the non-smoking comedian Roy Castle, whose lung cancer was said to arise from the time he had spent performing in smoky clubs. No such high-profile woman was presented as an 'innocent victim'. Research studies found that school children with parents who smoked received a significant dose—but mother's smoking had more impact than the father's. Soon 'passive smoking in utero' also appeared in the reports and cot deaths were linked with mothers who had smoked during pregnancy. At the same time a feminist turn in the public health coalition drew attention to the ways in which women were 'brainwashed' by mass advertising, a model which stressed the passivity of women and the way in which they were 'duped' by the industry's advertising tactics.[246] As we have seen in Chapter 8, this model of media effect ran counter to the conclusions of media theorists who argued that such effects were mediated and recalibrated in a more complex way.

But nevertheless, these developments meant that, once again, women were the main objects of fear and concern as they had been earlier for alcohol and for drugs. And, to add to that concern, a clear class divide had opened up in patterns of smoking and in the wake of the tax changes of the 1970s. This widened the gulf opening up between smokers and the mainstream of society. Health economists had argued in the 1970s that smoking was a waste of working-class life, and that higher taxes would prevent widening social inequality. But working-class smokers had remained resistant to higher prices for cigarettes and had continued to smoke. Research showed that people had accommodated to 'the facts' about smoking but there was a strong popular belief that the real risk from smoking was at the level of over twenty a day, a belief which had also emerged from research conducted in the 1950s. When researchers Alan Marsh and Stephen McKay published their book *Poor Smokers* in 1994, the debate opened up. It identified a clear group who were no longer the cultural norm. As Marsh commented, 'Thirty per cent of smokers are boxed up in the bottom ten per cent of income distribution.' 'Smoking', he said, was now 'the defiant badge of the underclass.'

Poor smokers were 'the last refuge of normative smoking. People here are still expected to smoke.'[247]

Women again bore the brunt of concern. The issue was increasingly defined as that of the smoking working-class lone mother. But not everyone agreed with this articulation. The sociologist Hilary Graham published research on lone mothers smoking in the late 1980s. Her attention was first drawn to this when women she was researching in the 1970s had been outraged by the Saatchi naked pregnant woman campaign. They resented the implication that they did not care, and also the naked model image. From Graham's interviews and the research diaries a different picture emerged, of smoking as an activity which gave order to chaotic and restricted days. Smoking was not just a way of structuring the women's caring for their children but also of reimposing order when structure broke down. 'It's the only thing I do for me', said one woman. Smoking was a way for poor mothers to cope. Graham drew attention to the paradoxical position of smoking for poor women. It contributed to a sense of wellbeing and promoted family welfare, while threatening physical health.[248] This research was not popular in public health circles. The sociologist Ann Oakley made a further point about the epidemiologically-based attack on women. If growth retardation in babies was due to foetal hypoxia, then why did this happen in some classes and not in others? Smoking in pregnancy had been singled out as a problem, but had not been seen as such when smoking was a cross-class activity. In classic public health terms, it was only when the problem was confined to the working class, and working-class women especially, that the rest of society began to fear it.

This fear and concern about a 'deviant minority' (although it was still large numerically) underpinned an overall change in culture and a new desire to regulate public space. Some legal cases brought smoking in the workplace on to the agenda, while safety concerns, in particular the Kings Cross fire of 1987, brought an end to smoking on the Underground in London. In 1988, British Airways ended smoking on domestic flights in the UK. New aircraft used recirculated air so smoking had to come to an end. It was a far cry from the

1970s when the British Airline Pilots Association (BALPA) had opposed proposals to ban pilots smoking in the cockpit.[249] At the end of the 1980s, Sir Peter Froggatt, the chair of the ISCSH during the 1980s commented on the significance of passive smoking in transforming the smoking question.

> The argument that smokers poison only themselves (or their unborn children?) can no longer be convincingly sustained. The conceptual framework within which government, industry, and the profession have worked, is fundamentally changed.[250]

That framework included public culture too. The science had given credibility to a process of marginalization of the smoker—and especially the smoking woman. Our factors of science, professionals, economics, and fear came into play to accelerate the marginalization of cigarettes from mainstream culture. Here was the beginning of a cultural 'tipping point' which we will follow in the succeeding chapters.

So far, this chapter has looked at the UK. As with alcohol and with drugs earlier, distinct national differences emerged in the way the issues—and the science—were responded to. In the United States, for example, although the core elements of the story were similar—the science of the 1950s (smoking and lung cancer, later heart disease) and the 1980s (passive smoking), responses were different. The role of the central state at the Federal level was less significant in the USA and this had important knock-on effects. For a start, the industry relationship with government was less corporatist than in the UK. Imperial had been a wartime partner of government and continued in that close role into the 1970s. It was only when changes of ownership occurred and the US companies entered the British market that relationships changed. Hence tobacco harm reduction had been a shared enterprise in the UK from the 1950s to the 1970s. But in the USA there was greater distance and a reliance on public relations strategies. Most of the major US companies had been spending significant sums on public relations and advertising since the early 1930s, tactics which were disliked by the British industry. The weakness of the state in the USA in health matters meant that some actions were taken at the Federal level—Congressional legislation to label packages and a ban on broadcast advertising—but much also happened through different routes. There were no national health education campaigns. Local action was important and also legal action—law suits which tried to apportion risk and blame. There was strong anti-industry emphasis in all of this and the culture of US society was much more strongly risk averse and was willing to accept locational constraints such as non-smoking restaurants earlier than in the UK, where there was more resistance to 'Puritanism'. As the US political scientist Constance Nathanson commented of the USA in the 1990s:

> The increasing political and legal vulnerability of the tobacco industry is part of a downward spiral, inseparable from concomitant changes in the number, composition, and social position of smokers. Thus, as the number of smokers in the population has declined to under 30 percent, as their composition has shifted towards younger and less affluent groups, and as adult smoking has become more and more stigmatized, it has become that much easier to attack the industry that supports the smoking habit.[251]

Other countries, in particular in Europe, did not follow the Anglo-American path, and Germany, for example, remained a country where smoking was still mainstream until quite recently.[252] An international dimension to the smoking issue started to emerge from the 1970s. Anti-smoking started to forge the sort of links which had marked the international temperance movement. Again, this formed part of more general developments in public health tactics and ideology. Public health as a movement was itself making significant strides at the international level in the 1970s and 1980s. The concepts of heath promotion and of primary health care were disseminated at the international level at that time. Primary health care emerged at Alma Ata in 1978 while health promotion emerged from the Canadian Lalonde Report in 1974, WHO's global strategy of *Health for All by the Year 2000* of 1981, and the *Ottawa Charter for Health Promotion* of 1986. Europe, too, emerged as a public health player with new policies on public health and directives on the subject which included tobacco in the late 1980s and early 1990s. Anti-tobacco coalitions developed at the European and international levels. The world conferences on tobacco which had started in the 1960s were an important initial vehicle for this. Ex CMO George Godber's speech at one in Norway in 1976 had a tone typical of the meetings as they developed:

> It's time to stop being gentle and persuasive with the merchants of death who make and sell these deadly things. Let's not ask for their cooperation—which we won't get—but tell them what their limits are.[253]

Australian influence was important as the Australian pioneered new anti-smoking and anti-industry tactics and some of the older international anti-TB networks reconfigured themselves to take on tobacco. Increasingly they looked to WHO to take on the issue. Moves for a global action plan on tobacco started in the 1980s. These went into decline under the director generalship of Nakajima in the late 1980s but revived strongly with a new focus on the international activities of the tobacco industry in the 1990s.

So by the late 1980s/early 1990s, the factors we identified at the outset of the book—science and its professionals, in this case public health epidemiologists; social movements; economics; fear; and internationalism—had combined to begin to push tobacco down a different path from the mass culture of the interwar years. Regulation varied from country to country, and, as with alcohol at the turn of the twentieth century, there were distinct cross-national differences in the way countries chose to respond to these public health facts. The Anglo-American and Northern European patterns of response were different to those in Southern Europe, with the exception of Germany in Northern Europe. But the interplay between regulation, culture, and science was there for all, although proceeding at a different national pace. Thresholds for public regulation and intervention were themselves social and political and in their turn both reflected and reacted upon culture. As smoking descended the social scale as a mainstream activity, the arguments against further regulation weakened still further.

10
Convergence or Divergence? Public Health and Neuroscience

Smoking, as we have seen, began to become detached from mainstream culture and to become a 'deviant' practice, a process which gathered pace from the 1980s. Anti-tobacco campaigners began to argue that, if tobacco had been discovered in the present, it would never have been a legal substance. Another debate, which rarely engaged with the tobacco discussions, was about whether drugs should be legalized or prohibited. In a sense both sets of arguments were beside the point. What such comments masked was a deeper issue. While commentators debated what *should* happen in the future, real change was taking place in the present. The substances were all engaged in a process of reconceptualization and repositioning which gathered pace towards the end of the twentieth century. These changes were not necessarily reflected in formal changes in regulation which reformers and activists urged, but there was nonetheless a reordering of boundaries. This chapter and the following one will look at those processes and how they built on some of the factors outlined earlier in the book. Were the substances converging to become more similar in the ways they were regulated and also used? Were responses to drug use becoming more liberal, while those to alcohol and smoking became more restrictive? Was everything now a 'drug'? The involvement of prescription, licit drugs, further complicated the picture. The forces at work were complex and could be leading to greater hedonism or to a more puritanical set of attitudes in society—both responses were possible.

This chapter will examine how drugs, alcohol, and tobacco (drugs and tobacco in particular) began to draw closer together in the second half of the twentieth century. It looks at the shifting of concepts and frameworks under the influence of different forms of science, as well as at practical outcomes in terms of treatment and other interventions. The overall argument stresses how substances began to fit within overall 'ways of looking' during this time. In particular the chapter will concentrate on

- The permeation of 'public health' ideas from tobacco to drugs and alcohol
- The realignment of 'disease' concepts across the substances
- The rise of harm reduction, in particular for drugs and for tobacco
- Treatment as an intervention and the rise of psychopharmacology as science.

New public health across the substances

Change began in the 1970s and accelerated towards the end of the twentieth century and in the early years of the twenty-first. Initially the effect was to move illicit drugs and tobacco towards a common framework; this chapter will look at that process. One key development was that the 'new public health' model, first applied to tobacco in the 1950s, began to extend across the substances. The public health model also began to extend from tobacco to drugs and to alcohol from the 1970s, the period when public health and primary care became central to international health initiatives. Drugs and alcohol retained elements of their earlier definition of 'disease', but new public health influences also became significant. The 'new public health' model also began to gain influence as part of the psychiatric model for drugs and alcohol in the 1970s.

Smoking had been reframed in this way from the 1950s: now alcohol and drugs were also subject to the same influences. Key crossover issues included the rise of 'whole population' theories of risk for alcohol consumption; the growing psychiatric interest in epidemiology as a research tool; and parallel adoption of these ideas in the drugs field. Both substances began to move away from an exclusively mental health way of looking.

As we saw earlier in the book, medical treatment for drug addiction and also for alcoholism was the model and these trends were in fact accentuated after the Second World War. Specialist alcohol treatment became part of the NHS in the 1950s and 1960s, while treatment for illicit drug use was located within general practice initially, and then the province of psychiatry. In the USA too, although slightly later, a national treatment system for drugs was developed in the wake of the Vietnam War. Returning servicemen who had become addicted while in Vietnam mostly managed to stop using drugs such as heroin on their return to a different setting. American researcher Lee Robins studied this group of returning servicemen and their changing patterns of drug use. She came to the conclusion that drug use was setting specific i.e. that it is not the outcome of a particular 'addictive personality' or a brain malfunction or an inherited disorder.[254] Servicemen who had used heroin in Vietnam had no problem in giving up that drug use once they returned home away from the war zone. What has often been overlooked in this discussion is the governmental response which went alongside it—the development by leading US drug psychiatrist Jerry Jaffe, drug czar under Richard Nixon, of a national treatment system dispensing methadone.[255] America, long the bastion of the 'war on drugs' approach and a prohibitionist response akin to that to alcohol in the 1920s, began to provide treatment and to develop its own 'medical model'.

But at the same time, public health approaches became important. Statistics and epidemiology were central to these new perceptions. Let us look at alcohol first. The French statistician Sully Ledermann had argued in the 1950s that there was a relationship between average per capita alcohol consumption and levels of alcohol misuse in a population. This theory had attracted little attention at the time, but in the 1970s it became central to what was termed a new public health approach to alcohol. This chimed also with population theories articulated by epidemiologists such as Geoffrey Rose in the public health field.

A new alcohol 'policy community' in the UK (the term used to characterize the interest groups and individuals focused on the substance) was led by psychiatrists but took on board civil servants, the alcohol voluntary sector, the police, and the law. Internationally this approach was articulated through the famous alcohol 'purple book' (called after the colour of its cover) *Alcohol Control Policies in Public Health Perspective* which was published in 1975 and jointly authored from the Finnish Foundation for Alcohol Studies, the Addiction Research Foundation in Toronto, and WHO Regional Office for Europe. Led by Kettil Bruun, a Finnish sociologist, and with a mix of social science and medical disciplines among its authors, the report cemented an alliance between psychiatry and a wider range of disciplines. Its influence can still be seen in the near present through the recent *Alcohol and the Public Good* and *Alcohol—No Ordinary Commodity*, produced by some members and descendants of the original team.[256] This new approach stressed that alcohol as an issue did not just comprise concern about the 'disease' of 'alcoholism', but that it was potentially a matter for everyone. Levels of drinking in the whole population were what mattered, not just the disease of a few.

In Britain, these public health ideas were presented in key reports to government in the late 1970s but did not find political approval with the change of government from Labour to Conservative in 1980. The electoral implications of seeing the electorate as a whole as 'the problem' were not lost on politicians. The epidemiological model of research also permeated into the alcohol and drugs field, in part because of the 'whole population' model for alcohol but also because of the interest of leading psychiatrists in US research where epidemiology was strong. The policy agenda too was becoming like that for smoking—restriction on advertising, monitoring, and self-control; higher taxation; and restriction of sale through licensing. This was the new public health agenda but it raised difficulties for politicians who had the electoral implications in mind.

The drugs field was also affected by public health ideas. Again, these were part of more traditional psychiatric and clinical responses. Key changes in policy took place in the 1960s. The changes were much debated, as those of Rolleston in the 1920s had been. The main change was the replacement of the general practitioner, sometimes in private practice, as the main source of expertise, by a psychiatric specialist hospital-based system. Concern had been expressed in the late 1950s and early 1960s about the operation of the GP system. One doctor in particular, Lady Isabella Frankau, working in Harley Street, was prescribing large amounts of heroin and cocaine to addicts. In 1962, she prescribed a total of 6 kilograms (600,000 tablets) of heroin. On one occasion, she prescribed 9 grams (900 tablets) of heroin to an addict and gave the same patient a further 6 grams (600 tablets) three days later to replace pills lost in an accident. Frankau and a small number of other doctors working in NHS general practice were thought to be overprescribing heroin and other drugs to addicts. Concern within the Ministry of Health, and the rising numbers of addicts (although these were still very small) led to the reconvening in 1964 of the interdepartmental committee on heroin addiction (the Brain Committee) under the chairmanship of Sir Russell Brain, a neurologist and former president of the Royal College of Physicians. Brain had chaired a previous committee on the same subject which had reported in 1961 and had reaffirmed the Rolleston position.[257] The Brain report which was published in 1965 saw the establishment of specialist treatment centres (Drug Dependence Units—DDUs) under psychiatric leadership and the removal of responsibility for prescription from the GP. Doctors outside the DDUs were still able to prescribe heroin for pain relief but not for patients who were addicted to the drug.

The change in the balance of expertise was dependent on a new view of addiction and its treatment, and this is where public health ideas came in. No longer was this simply an issue between the individual doctor and patient, but the issue also assumed a clear social dimension as well. The committee recommended that those seeking treatment for addiction be notified to a central authority, as was the case for infectious disease. But in this case, the central authority was the Home Office, not the Ministry of Health, thus reaffirming the medico-penal concordat contained within policy since the 1920s. The definition of addiction itself changed to encompass a view of social infection—'for addiction is a socially infectious condition and its notification may offer a means for epidemiological assessment and control'. Clinics were to control the spread of addiction into the wider population and also treat the individual addict. Here was an emergent alliance between older and newer forms of public health and psychiatric concepts. The Brain Committee's concept of the potential 'social infection' of drug addiction proposed epidemiological assessment and control. Brain's formulation significantly encapsulated older traditions of public health—infection control and notification of disease—with newer ones: risk, epidemiology, and the potential 'infection' of the whole population with drug addiction.

A model of dealing with drugs which combined psychiatry and mental health with public health styles emerged in the 1960s. This also infiltrated research, which was developing in this period. There were epidemiological surveys of drug users in local areas. The Americans were developing what was called 'community epidemiology' in the drugs field and its influence filtered into the UK. In the 1980s local studies of drug use became key to policymaking using epidemiological methods of capture/recapture to try to estimate user numbers.[258]

To sum up, then, the psychiatric and public health models moved closer together in the 1970s for our chosen substances. But the professional groupings were still distinct. Psychiatrists were the lead figures for alcohol and drugs. The public health smoking field was located in public health epidemiology and was wedded to individual self-help, behavioural modification, and abstention as its aims.

Later in the century a crisis took the public health stance further for drugs. The advent of HIV/AIDS in the 1980s was the catalyst. In the late

1970s and early 1980s, the psychiatric-run clinics had aimed to restrict prescribing and to get addicts off drugs within a defined period of time. This was a tactic which was justified by research, a controlled trial of injectable heroin versus oral methadone consumption as treatment modalities. The results of the trial were equivocal, but methadone was assessed as a more challenging treatment—even though it might lead to greater involvement in the black market as addicts turned there for the heroin they really wanted. But it gave the research results which clinic staff wanted. They hoped for a more therapeutic function rather than long-term drug dispensing to addicts who did not move on. A groundswell of opposition to this policy had developed among other interests in the drug field, including some psychiatrists and the drugs voluntary sector most notably. But such opposition had no political pull. The new Conservative government in the 1980s was initially closely wedded to a US-style 'war on drugs' approach.

The coming of HIV/AIDS changed all that. The threat that HIV/AIDS might spread into the general population through the conduit of drug use enabled a new public health response to drugs to be articulated. This came about initially in 1986 because of the situation among drug users in Scotland, where the virus had spread rapidly in Edinburgh. The 1986 McClelland Report on HIV/AIDS and drugs concluded:

> There is…a serious risk that infected drug misusers will spread HIV beyond the presently recognized high-risk groups and into the sexually active general population. Very extensive spread by heterosexual contacts has already occurred in a number of African countries…There is…an urgent need to contain the spread of HIV infection among drug misusers not only to limit the harm caused to drug misusers themselves but also to protect the health of the general public. The gravity of the problem is such that on balance the containment of the spread of the virus is a higher priority in management than the prevention of drug misuse.[259]

These words later informed an influential report published by the English Advisory Council on the Misuse of Drugs in 1988. The new public health approach for drugs involved the expansion of treatment, the provision of needle exchange, and the prescription of methadone, the substitute opiate. From the late 1980s onwards this 'new dawn' of drug treatment was widely promoted in the UK. HIV/AIDS did not have the same public health impact on the drug field in the USA, where concern among ethnic groups about the potential 'genocide' involved in the provision of needles to black drug users brought an opposition which was absent in the UK.

So by the 1980s/90s the frameworks around drugs and alcohol had changed to accommodate public health ideas and to make them a more central part of the discourse. Public health epidemiological research and ideas about 'risk' and 'the population' had permeated both fields.

The realignment of disease concepts

Another development which saw movement and repositioning was the reordering of concepts and ideas about the nature of the underlying disorder. Concept shift took place with new ideas about 'use' and 'problem use' applied to illicit drugs, while, conversely, drug-focused ideas of 'addiction' began to be applied to tobacco. Tobacco was changing places to become more like a drug, while drug use itself was becoming 'normalized' and part of a wide spectrum of substance use in society. From the 1980s onward, new ideas about drug use tended to see it as more 'normal' while tobacco smoking became seen as pathological. One of the interesting aspects of this change was the interim history of an attempt in the 1970s to unify the substances through the concept of 'dependence', which failed but was the precursor of changes towards the end of the century.

In the earlier chapters of the book, we saw that alcohol and drugs had developed a quite distinct conceptual framing to that of tobacco. The model was one of disease, which had justified treatment. Addiction had developed from about the time of the First World War as the model for drugs in particular, emerging from the earlier inebriety model. Addiction had never been as strong for alcohol during those years but a 'disease model' of 'alcoholism' had revived for alcohol in the 1930s.

A new scientific understanding of alcohol developed in the post pro-hibitionist USA. The scientist E. M. Jellinek, who later transferred to the newly established WHO in the 1950s, and led its focus on alcohol there, became head of a multidisciplinary research programme on the invitation of Howard W. Haggard, head of the Laboratory of Applied Physiology at Yale University. The influence of Jellinek, Yale, the *Quarterly Journal of Studies on Alcohol* which they founded, and Yale summer schools, filtered into the UK, where it appealed to leading psychiatrists. The rediscovery of disease was what had lain behind the involvement of psychiatry in alcoholism treatment in the 1950s and 1960s. Such concepts were legitimated and given authority in the postwar world by the definitions adopted by WHO. In the 1960s the Brain Committee had used the definition of addiction produced by WHO's expert committee on addiction producing drugs which had reported in 1957. It was a 'state of periodic or chronic intoxication produced by the repeated consumption of a drug' and was a form of mental illness, not criminal behaviour. The definition distinguished 'addiction' from 'habit'.

In the 1960s and 1970s, however, ideas about disease had shifted at international, and subsequently at national levels and there were possi-bilities at that time of the substances being conceptualized in a com-mon framework. A new word, 'dependence', was introduced to categorize what had previously been called 'addiction'. WHO's expert committee had proposed in 1965 that the term 'drug dependence' should be used instead of addiction in order to clarify existing termi-nology. But this was more than a simple clarification. The older term had seemed to place too much emphasis on the physical effects of addiction whereas the new one brought more psychological under-standings into play. It dropped the biomedical overtones of addiction in favour of newer personality oriented approaches. Such concepts were not 'value free' or simple expressions of progress in scientific understanding. They were the outgrowth of scientific alliances and also served to reinforce them. Dependence was a term which was widely used in the drugs field in the 1970s. It was defined as 'a state arising from repeated administration of a drug on a periodic or continuous basis', with characteristics which varied according to the type of drug involved. It could be 'psychic and sometimes physical'. The newly established Advisory Committee, later the ACMD, was originally called the Advisory Committee on Drug Dependence (ACDD). The newly established drug information organization of this period was called the Institute for the Study of Drug Dependence (ISDD). The use of the term reflected the alliance on the ground and in research between psychiatry and psychology.

For alcohol, which was seen at the time as occupying an intermediate position between habit-forming and addiction-producing drugs, new concepts involving dependence were elaborated in 1977—the 'alcohol dependence syndrome' and 'alcohol related disabilities', the former again combining physical and psychological dependence and the latter developed, according to the social scientist Robin Room, to support US drives for reimbursable treatment under insurance cover.[260] And the concept also filtered into the tobacco field. The 1971 report of the Royal College of Physicians on smoking had a section on 'the smoking habit' which had discussion of motivation and psychology, including Freudian explanation and the roles of personality and inheritance. But it also noted that some craved nicotine and that what it called 'dependent smokers' needed special clinics.[261] Such changing definitions were part of WHO's International Classification of Disease (ICD), the 'bible' of agreed cross-national definitions of disease. A category of dependence for smoking was added in 1974.

Dependence as a concept thus had the ability to unify the substance field in the 1970s. It was being applied to some extent across the substances. But it largely failed to bring them closer together conceptually at that stage. The reason lay in strategic issues and the position of actors on the ground, in particular the strength of the public health focus on self-determination, lifestyle change, and abstention as the ultimate aim. The tobacco field did not embrace psychiatry and other components of the alcohol/drugs treatment arena. In fact, in England, the psychiatrist Michael Russell, who ran the smoking programme at the London Institute of Psychiatry's Addiction Research Unit (ARU), was an unpopular figure in public health anti-smoking circles. He was a strong advocate of 'dependence' as a concept and harm reduction, using nicotine, as a strategy. The attempt to do this at the ARU was an early harbinger of later 'addiction'-focused moves which brought the substances together from the 1990s.

The psychologists working on alcohol at this time were focused on harm reduction, for ideas about 'controlled drinking' were influential in the 1970s. But the smoking field aimed to work towards abstention, an objective which had been strengthened after the failure of safer smoking and new smoking material initiatives of the decade. A paper written by Russell in 1971 stated that 'cigarette smoking is probably the most addictive and dependence producing form of object specific self-administered gratification known to man' and his overall stance on dependence remained isolated from the mainstream public health anti-smoking field.

In the 1980s and 1990s conceptual shifts continued and to some degree alcohol drugs and smoking moved closer together under the banner of the new psychological focus on behaviour change which undercut the model of dependence. Developments within psychology focused on what was called the 'attitude model' and the development of 'affect control' was seen as of crucial importance. The new directions gave greater prominence to the public health tactic of health education, but this was education which did not stress damage (which simply made smokers fatalistic) but rather the health benefits of giving up. Smoking for psychologists became a case study of the wider issue of behaviour change with the models also applied to drugs and to alcohol. The work of US psychologists Prochaska and Di Clemente was of great significance. A psychologist commented, 'Psychologists became less linked to treatment. There's less emphasis on clinical approaches and more on community and public health.'[263]

Further developments brought incipient alliances around another new concept—that of 'problem' use. This formulation began to be applied to both drugs and alcohol from the 1980s. This took the 'habit' and 'disability' component of previous theoretical discussions of addiction/dependence and reformulated them as problem alcohol or problem drug use. The term appeared in the ACMD's report on *Treatment and Rehabilitation* which was published in 1982. There, a problem drug taker was defined as 'any person who experiences social, psychological, physical, or legal problems related to intoxication and/or regular excessive consumption and/or dependence as a consequence of his own use of drugs or other chemical substances (excluding alcohol or tobacco)'.[264] Although alcohol was specifically excluded in the definition, the same concept had already been applied to alcohol as well. There, the concept took off in the late 1960s and was elaborated in Don Cahalan's 1970 book *Problem Drinkers*. It gained additional purchase from the consumption/harm public health perspective of the alcohol 'purple book'. In the mid 1970s in the UK a short-lived Advisory Council on Alcoholism had stressed the importance of reaching different groups of 'problem drinkers', many of whom could not be reached using a treatment approach. Such reformulations also reflected the involvement of a wider range of health and other personnel in the management of these substances. The voluntary sector, social workers, police, and probation workers were all involved, as well as specialist psychiatrists. Again, the reformulation encompassed a wider range of users of the substances, but did not quite encompass tobacco. For the tobacco field, all users were the problem, rather than a particular group for whom use was a problem.

After these earlier attempts at conceptual alliance, the concept which ultimately served to bring about a closer alignment between the substances was, perhaps surprisingly, that of 'addiction'. Tobacco use began to be seen as a form of addiction. This book argues that this was not simply a dawning of scientific understanding but rather a 'fact waiting to happen', that is a scientific fact with implications which energized alliances within the tobacco field. The concept of addiction had, as we have seen, never been central to tobacco discourse. There was a potential conflict over what the model implied for the public health approach. One interviewee summed up the conflict between public health and psychiatric models. It was a matter of what the concept implied and also the institutional and professional location of the message.

> By establishing the efficacy of nicotine replacement we're moving towards the public health model of brief interventions in primary care. That's a more acceptable message that has filtered through... Nicotine is less acceptable. People found it difficult to accept it as a form of drug addiction. They felt it was counter productive to label it as an addiction because it absolved people from responsibility... the association with the Maudsley was a problem—it wasn't a mental health issue[265]

Addiction initially had been in conflict with the dominant public health agenda for tobacco; and the location of its primary advocate in a psychiatric setting compounded the problems with its acceptability in the public health field.

In the 1990s the rise of the 'new' arena of psychopharmacology and the re-importation of these ideas from the United States, gave them a new life in the smoking arena. Psychopharmacology as a discipline was of course not new in the UK or elsewhere. Its early development had been in relation to psychiatry in the years between the 1940s and 1960s with the rise of the amphetamines, the use of LSD in the treatment of mental illness and the rise of the benzodiazepines.[266] Such developments were far from the epidemiological interests of the public health field of the period, which was consciously moving away from the 'medical model'. For tobacco and its incipient alliance with illicit drugs the crucial development was work at Aberdeen by John Hughes and Hans Kosterlitz, the discovery of the opiate receptors in the mid 1970s, and the pharmacological impact this had on concepts of addiction. Hughes wrote in the late 1980s:

> The pharmacological approach to addiction in its broadest sense involves the use of drugs as tools to probe all aspects of tolerance and dependence, and inevitably overlaps with the behavioural approach. Over recent years cooperation between pharmacologists, biochemists and psychologists with new theories has led to major advances towards defining the neural substrates for various dependent related processes. These advances in psychopharmacology build on the premise that it is

the rewarding or reinforcing consequences of drug action which are responsible for the initiation and maintenance of drug abuse.[267]

The concept of addiction was reimported from the USA where there had been an expansion of work in psychopharmacology since the 1970s. Murray Jarvik's group at Albert Einstein College in New York, which had worked on the effects of drugs on animals and on memory, turned its attention to work on nicotine in the early 1970s. The project was supported by the American Cancer Society which had not funded basic pharmacology before. There had been little nicotine research in the USA—it was not a popular area. A US researcher remembered,

> It was seen as not being a proper drug-interest in opiate dependence was rising...people were interested in nicotine pharmacology—there were those who felt nicotine was an old drug and the basic pharmacology had been investigated. Others saw that nothing was known about the role of nicotine in smoking. There were parallels with cannabis but studies there were impeded by the lack of an active principle—it was difficult to do good laboratory work.[268]

Work by Goldstein and others at Stanford brought work on morphine, heroin, and methadone together with that on nicotine and caffeine.[269]

What led to this change of stance in the tobacco field and what caused such ideas to be acceptable? Here, two sets of explanations have been in play. One stresses the standard 'march of scientific understanding', i.e. that scientific discovery enabled addiction to be identified whereas previously it had not. The advent of psychopharmacology in this field was what mattered. The other explanation is a more conspiratorial one—that the 'fact' of addiction had been well known to the tobacco companies but they had kept it quiet. Hence no one had talked about addiction because they did not know of it. The image supporting this argument and known to many is that of the chief executives of American tobacco companies, hands raised and declaring on oath before a congressional committee in 1994 that tobacco was not addictive. Shortly after this the UCSF anti-tobacco activist Stanton Glantz was sent tobacco industry documents which showed that one tobacco industry executive had been aware that cigarettes were addictive back in 1963. The industry had funded research which had shown this decades before. The whole exposé was later filmed as 'The Insider'. So the public discussion of the concept of addiction for smoking has been dominated by this 'heroes and villains' tale of a 'hidden concept' concealed by the duplicity of the tobacco industry.

That is certainly part of the US story but, in reality, the 'rise of addiction' as a key concept for smoking in different national locations from the 1980s/90s was a much more complex affair. Neither 'march of progress' nor 'conspiracy' models quite help fully to explain it. It also had much to do with changes in the strategies of public health and with new scientific alliances emerging at this time, and, in the UK, with political change in the 1990s and the aims of the incoming Labour government. The rise and fall of concepts owes much to these changing contextual circumstances and alliances. We have stressed earlier how the concept of dependence reflected the interests of new scientific alliances in the field, as did that of 'problem' use. The same was the case for addiction and smoking later on. As we have seen, the dominant public health ideology in the 1970s was based on ideas about self-control and abstinence. It was not the case that public health people were unaware of addiction but rather that the concept had no meaning or significance because of the way public health was focused at the time.

Research on nicotine habituation in the UK had started in the 1960s in the industry's own joint laboratories, based in Harrogate in Yorkshire and organized by the cross industry Tobacco Research Council. The work was part of the aim at that time of finding out what was harmful about tobacco and the eventual removal of the harmful components. Alongside mice experiments, work on nicotine was developed, work which was presented at major symposia and published in *Nature* in the late 1960s.[270,271] The Harrogate research was widely cited in the emergent scientific field of pharmacology and can hardly be said to have been secret. In fact, it was presented in April–May 1967 to members of the RCP committee on smoking, and advice was sought on the balancing of tar and nicotine in cigarettes because of the issue of habit. The industry did not want to develop cigarettes which did not sell because the nicotine content was too low.[273]

Public health researchers did know, but the fact was not important when the agenda and tactics were elsewhere. In the 1980s and 1990s the stance changed. Despite the revelations about 'passive smoking', smokers still proved stubbornly unwilling to give up and, as we have seen, smoking was becoming concentrated in the lower—and female—sections of the population. How could this be understood and dealt with in policy terms? Addiction provided one answer. Product modification came back onto the agenda, in part through the work of the government's Independent Scientific Committee on Smoking and Health, which did major work on nicotine and its role in the 1980s. A report from the Committee in 1984 drew attention to the role of nicotine in maintaining smoking as a habit. In 1986 the chair of the committee, Sir Peter Froggatt, and the researcher Nicholas Wald summarized key results. The evidence showed that nicotine levels should be brought down, but that the toxicity of cigarettes would be reduced more if tar came down more than nicotine. They recognized addiction as a double edged issue. It was a reason to maintain nicotine levels in cigarettes (to make them less harmful) or to lower them in order to wean people off the habit.[274] This work marked a major repositioning and it mattered that, although the work was funded at arm's length by the tobacco industry, the researchers were untainted by industry associations. The research also marked a rapprochement in scientific styles between epidemiological approaches and those of psychopharmacology. This was part of a more general trend in public health research. These years also saw changes within the science of public health, where stand-alone epidemiological approaches were criticized and a greater rapprochement occurred with different modes including toxicology and biomedicine.

In 1988 a US Surgeon General's report on nicotine addiction was important in giving the concept the stamp of approval and the UK RCP published its report *Nicotine Addiction in Britain* in 2000. But the responses in the two countries differed. In the USA the Food and Drug Administration (FDA) tried to get nicotine under its aegis as a 'drug' and declared it to be addictive. The idea in the US was that levels of nicotine would be reduced, which was the not the case in the UK. Snowdon argues that the fact of 'addiction' was already known, but class actions had less chance of success if juries believed that the addictive power of nicotine was long-standing common knowledge.[275] Certainly the industry's opposition began to crumble in the late 1990s and a number of class actions were settled with large compensation sums. The US industry had been lowering levels of both tar and nicotine since the 1960s. But the concept of 'helpless addiction' gave a clear argument for the anti-tobacco forces to use against the industry's argument that smokers did it out of free will.

At the same time as the smoker was being reconceptualized as a helpless addict, the drug addict was being redefined as a self-confident 'user' with rights in the provision of services. In April 2006 a group of drug user activists from around the world met at the 17th International Conference on the Reduction of Drug Related Harm in Vancouver, Canada. Together they produced a statement essentially of drug users' rights:

> We are people from around the world who use drugs. We are people who have been marginalized and discriminated against; we have been killed, harmed unnecessarily, put in jail, depicted as evil, and stereotyped as dangerous and disposable. Now it is time to raise our voices as citizens, establish our rights and reclaim the right to be our own spokespersons striving for self-representation and self-empowerment.[276]

Groups of drug users came together as activists, as service users, and as carer groups, and in the UK were given a greater role in the formulation of service policy. There were complaints that such involvement was only tokenistic, and indeed that was often the case. But the concept of 'the user' was significant, for it replaced the idea of the passive 'addict' and recipient of services with a much more active concept. In a sense the tobacco 'user' had become the 'addict' while the drug 'addict' had become the 'user'.

Harm reduction as a common concept and approach

However, tactics considered appropriate to deal with both began to demonstrate overlap. One tactic—harm reduction—became common to all substances and in particular for illicit drugs and tobacco in the

1980s and 1990s. Harm reduction was initially a controversial concept in British drug policy, widely supported in the drug voluntary sector and among health interests but with no purchase at the policy level. Conservative politicians remained wedded officially to the 'war on drugs' approach in the early 1980s. The advent of HIV/AIDS enabled such ideas to move into the realm of practical policy. Key civil servants in the Department of Health worked with researchers evaluating needle exchange initiatives to ensure that the feasibility of harm reduction tactics was presented to ministers as an effective strategy.[277] Harm reduction was initially a policy strategy aimed at the reduction of HIV/AIDS and the prevention of its spread into the general population. In the 1990s, under the incoming Labour government, it became allied to a criminal justice agenda. The argument was that harm reduction tactics would reduce the prison population. The subsequent coalition government policy focused more on the idea of 'recovery', moving the user towards a drug-free life rather than maintenance on methadone. So harm reduction as a tactic appeared in 2012 to be less prominent for drugs than it had been, although the guidelines for treatment adopted under the previous harm reduction regimes continued to operate and professionals in the field were discussing whether recovery was a process which could also encompass 'stages of change'.

Harm reduction also came into play for tobacco and this tactic became an international debate at the turn of the twentieth and twenty-first centuries. The rise of the concept of nicotine addiction in the USA led to a process of 'stamping out addiction', much as Americans had tried to do with drugs in the 1920s. In 2012, the American historian Robert Proctor published a book significantly entitled *Golden Holocaust* in which he advocated a move to a prohibitionist regime, one which would be underpinned by FDA regulation of nicotine levels.[278] In the UK, nicotine addiction as a 'scientific fact' led to different responses. Law suits were not an important tactic for public health researchers as they were in the USA and the policy framework within which smoking operated was different. The 'fact' of addiction led instead to a revived focus on 'harm reduction' for smoking. If smokers were addicted and it was proving impossible for them to give up, then at least they should be given a clean product. This had been Russell's argument since the 1970s but he had then gained little support. In a powerful 1991 editorial in the *Lancet*, he argued the case for nicotine maintenance:

> What distinguishes nicotine from other widely abused drugs is that its effects are subtle and do not cause socially disruptive intoxication, provoke violence, or impair performance. Yet deaths due to tobacco far outnumber those caused by all other drugs. The central paradox is that, while people smoke for nicotine, they die mainly from the tar and other unwanted components in the smoke. Why have governments persisted in allowing the manufacture, extensive advertising, and promotion of such a lethally contaminated drug delivery system as the cigarette, while putting so little pressure on the tobacco industry to develop more purified forms of nicotine delivery?[279]

In the early twenty-first century, some public health interests changed their position on harm reduction. The Health Education Authority, usually a bastion of mainstream public health sentiment, published a report on regulating nicotine delivery systems, and innovations from the tobacco industry (the smokeless cigarette and nicotine delivery devices) led to calls for a nicotine regulatory authority which would provide an overall regulatory umbrella. The argument was similar to that made for methadone maintenance for drug addicts. Nicotine replacement therapy (NRT) became a central plank of the government's strategy against inequality. Sir Donald Acheson, the former Chief Medical Officer, chaired a government enquiry into inequality and declared that NRT was one of the top three most effective ways of dealing with inequality. Leading tobacco researchers in the UK began to call for more effective harm reduction tactics. In 2011 researchers at the Centre for Tobacco Control Studies at the University of Nottingham drew attention to the fact that tobacco control policy was too limited. It focused on preventing young people from starting to smoke and getting current smokers to quit. They commented:

> many smokers cannot or do not want to give up, and little effort has been put into reducing the harmfulness of their continued tobacco

use ... The sooner the action starts and the less hazardous the product is, the greater the harm reduction.[280]

The problems in fully establishing the approach were that nicotine replacement products were marketed as cessation aids, not as longer-term substitutes for smoking. There was a need to make them at a dosage and form of delivery which was acceptable as a substitute for cigarettes. Accessibility and affordability were also issues. Snus, a smokeless tobacco, which was said to have contributed to declining smoking prevalence in Sweden, was banned elsewhere in Europe under existing regulatory systems. In 2011, there were growing calls for a European tobacco and nicotine regulatory authority which would regulate the substances in a more rational way with regard to actual harms. This position remained deeply controversial within the tobacco public health community. It raised concerns that people might be recruited to smoking by the availability of lower hazard tobacco products; about the long-term health risks of some products; and about the implications of 'supping with the devil', about collaboration with 'the industry', whether pharmaceutical or tobacco.[281] It was notable too that little research had been done in these areas. In 2013, the European Parliament was seeking urgently to fund research on electronic cigarettes, which were later classified as medicines.[282] Given the history of past collaboration, such tactics seemed to be less controversial in the UK than in the USA. There was initially surprisingly little cross-fertilization between 'harm reductionists' in the drug field and for tobacco.

Treatment as a public health intervention and the rise of psychopharmacology

The nature of harm reduction in practice was also similar for drugs and tobacco, for medication became a form of prevention, a development which was in line with wider trends in public health at that time. And science, too, provided another universalizing mechanism, with the ideas of epidemiology applied to drugs and to alcohol in the 1970s, drawing on the public health model, while brain science and psychopharmacology became a further form of universalizing scientific model across the substances from the 1990s.

Public health and treatment became synonymous in some cases. For drugs, the response was one based on technology (the syringe) and also on the provision of a medicine, in the form of methadone. Methadone was key. This synthetic opiate was first isolated in the late 1930s, and was both cheaper and with longer lasting action than heroin. The prescription of the drug had became common in the clinics in the 1970s during and after the controlled trial: it represented more 'active' treatment and fitted better with professional aspirations for a more therapeutic relationship with addicts. In the 1980s, methadone was redefined again, not as a substitute for heroin this time, but as both a treatment and a preventive public health strategy. Prescribing the drug could attract addicts who would otherwise go to the black market or indulge in unsafe injecting practices, into treatment and health services. The aim was firstly to curb the spread of HIV into the general population, the 'infection' model which had also been articulated by the Brain committee more than thirty years before. Its use was followed by a wider range of pharmaceutical interventions such as Subutex (buprenorphine), licensed for the treatment of addiction in Britain in 1999 and also the use of full opioid agonists such as Naltrexone which blocked the effect of heroin on the addicts brain altogether, approved by NICE for use in 2007. Public health approaches and pharmaceutical interventions became to some extent synonymous.

The public health methadone model—of treatment as prevention and the provision of pharmaceuticals—was a more general trend in the public health field in these decades. One parallel was with the prescription of statins for the prevention of heart disease after trials in the 1980s and 1990s. Prescription of statins rocketed in the late twentieth century. Statins were thought to be taken by one in three people over forty. Up to seven million people in England were taking them in 2011, costing the NHS at least £450 million a year. There was criticism of this approach with the argument that the NHS was spending huge amounts of money in medicating large sections of the population. It was an international approach too and the American historian Jeremy Greene has pointed to the alignment from the 1960s between public health and the pharmaceutical industry in the treatment/prevention of asymptomatic disease states.[283]

For tobacco, too, treatment became a public health tactic and so contributed to the shifting of substance boundaries. Treatment, as we saw in earlier chapters of the book, had played little of a role in the earlier 'new public health' approach to tobacco. Epidemiology and individual behaviour change were key, utilizing the techniques of mass media persuasion. Any treatment model was very weakly established. A number of anti-smoking clinics had been set up in the wake of the Doll Hill research and the RCP 1962 report but they were staffed mainly by psychologists rather than doctors. Therapy was based on psychological theories of learned behaviour. Hypnosis, aversion therapy, rapid smoking, and 'satiation' all had their advocates, and there were walk-in clinics and group therapy. Later, in the late 1970s, the rise of primary health care and the emphasis on the role of the general practitioner saw attention paid to his or her role in a 'brief intervention', advice on giving up smoking or moderating alcohol use. But the idea of treatment in general did not fit well with the ideology of public health, which stressed self-control and the role of the individual in securing good health. The anti-tobacco public health activist Simon Chapman attacked the idea of treatment because of its doctor focus and in general the public health movement from the 1970s saw abstinence through self-control as the answer, not medicine.

In fact, there was no 'treatment' as such at this time and the 'brief intervention' research relied instead on the personality of the doctor. The early research which supported this approach had been carried out for alcohol by Griffith Edwards, a psychiatrist recognized to have strong personal magnetism.[284] Primary care had no treatment to offer. Then new technology opened up a new avenue. The development of NRT through the Swedish pharmaceutical industry and its association with researchers at the Institute of Psychiatry offered a route to medicalization and treatment. Here was the 'medicine' which smoking had lacked.

The British drug regulation body, the Committee on the Safety of Medicines (CSM) licensed nicotine chewing gum in 1980 for general use as an anti-smoking aid, a decision based on the usual grounds of safety and efficacy. But another committee in the regulatory structures, the significantly titled Advisory Committee on Borderline Substances, ruled out its use in NHS prescriptions because of doubts about efficacy. NRT was for a while in the difficult position of being the only prescription-based medicine which was not available on the NHS. A doctor who did write such a prescription was brought in front of an NHS tribunal. Further change came in the 1990s as some nicotine products moved into the over-the-counter (OTC) category, meaning that they could be sold under pharmaceutical supervision. With the election of the Labour government in 1997, NRT assumed much greater importance as an aid for stopping smoking but also as a form of maintenance treatment. NRT was switched to the general sales category and promoted as an intervention which would help narrow the inequalities gap. For a while it was free to those on low incomes. A 2005 working party of the CSM recommended NRT to be licensed for adolescents, pregnant and breast-feeding women, and smokers with cardiovascular and other underlying diseases; and saw NRT as a maintenance drug. Some products were licensed to cut down smoking as a 'stepping stone' to stopping completely, for smokers who were currently unable to stop abruptly.[285] NRT had become like methadone and other 'public health treatments', both treatment and long-term maintenance drug.

Medication became the public health tactic but it also seemed appropriate because of another scientific development at the end of the century. Psychopharmacology was a powerful mode of repositioning and bringing them into a common framing. The language of addiction had been re-emergent for the other substances since the 1980s. It was 'in the air' more generally. This emergence came from a number of different scientific directions. Of particular importance—and providing a symbolic link between disease and public health arenas—was the use of theories of addiction in the health economics field. Gary Becker's theory of 'rational addiction' elaborated in a 1988 paper had argued that addiction was an economically rational act.[286] But the argument from brain science was the one which gained most purchase in the USA. Alan Leshner, the head of the American drugs agency NIDA (National Institute on Drug Abuse) declared in a 1997 article in *Science*, where he reviewed the past twenty years of research, that addiction was a 'chronic relapsing brain disorder'. The subtext for this stance in the USA was a more liberal attitude, a more compassionate view of drugs and addiction, the promotion of a physiological view which appeared to be 'value free' and would underpin the idea of addicts as patients to be treated, rather than as objects caught up in the 'war on drugs'. As the historian Tim Hickman has pointed out, post 9/11, this liberal ethos changed. The idea of the 'hijacked brain' gained new resonance. Public health was a movable feast subject to many redefinitions. After 9/11, in particular in the USA, it redefined itself round the fight against terrorism, another 'threat from without'; thus the original strategy of the promoters of the idea for drugs was lost.[287]

But psychopharmacology did bring the substances together, not least through its powerful visual representations of the addicted brain. The brain of the compulsive cocaine user did not look that different to the brain of individuals addicted to nicotine. As Hickman has pointed out, these were highly stylized representations which were not objectively 'real'. Nor was the relationship between this mapping and actual behaviour clear. In Britain, the brain science agenda dominated the government's Foresight initiative on addiction and society in 2007. The government's chief scientific adviser Sir David King welcomed the results of the initiative and underlined the blurring of boundaries between list and illicit drugs which Foresight foretold:

> The greatest changes we will see in the twenty-first century may be brought to us through developments in our understanding of the brain. These advances may offer revolutionary treatments for the brain, and could see the end of neuro-degenerative disorders such as Alzheimer's and Parkinson's diseases. We should also see much improved treatments for addiction and other mental health disorders, and the development of new recreational drugs some of which might lead to fewer harms and lower risks of addiction than the substances in use today.[288]

For various reasons, these scientific developments put some social scientists, usually quick to declaim the 'social construction' of such ideas, on the back foot. In the UK historians debated whether the new brain science could be accommodated, rather than deconstructed. Some US historians also claimed that this was science which should be taken seriously: the US historian of drugs, David Courtwright, advised fellow historians to 'take a hit of neuroscience'.[289] Such historians had never positioned themselves within the sociology of scientific knowledge field and so their acceptance of the 'value free' nature of new scientific ideas was not surprising. An alternative historical approach, that taken here, is to examine the role these new formulations played in research and in policy and the clusters of influence which supported them. The psychologist Stanton Peele, an opponent of theories of addiction in general, called the new developments 'high-tech phrenology'. Nonetheless, in the USA the brain disease model gained priority for government research funding and in the UK also, the MRC's addiction initiative funded a good deal of this sort of work.

So the postwar years saw a period of repositioning of the substances in terms of the ways in which they were conceptualized and the sciences and approaches which were central. Partnerships between traditional 'new public health' sciences and neuroscience were more common by the early twenty-first century and the role of psychiatry was less prominent for alcohol and for drugs than it had been in the 1950s and 1960s. But public health itself changed and became focused on pharmaceutical interventions, on treatment as prevention as well as cure. This stress on the pharmaceutical was a more general tendency which we will examine in the next chapter and which served to bring a wider range of medicines and drugs into the equation. Smoking and drugs, tobacco/nicotine and heroin/methadone were repositioning from the 1980s. This chapter has mainly focused on those two substances. As we will see in the final chapter, there are more recent signs that alcohol, too, is beginning to move and reposition under the impetus of some of the forces identified through the earlier chapters of the book.

11
Hedonism or Control?

The repositioning of substances brought illicit drugs and tobacco closer together: tobacco, which in British government medicines regulation had been classified as a 'borderline substance'—i.e. neither clearly medicine nor drug, or even food—was in the process of aligning with the idea of an illicit drug. Alcohol initially remained separate from these developments, although the British government's first alcohol strategy, published in 2004 was the Alcohol Harm Reduction Strategy on the model of drug harm reduction. Although public health researchers categorized it as 'our favourite drug', it retained its position as a culturally sanctioned and regulated intoxicating substance. But in the early twenty-first century its location also began to change; alcohol began a process of repositioning that in some respects was consciously modelled, by reforming interests, on the route already taken by tobacco. This chapter examines the shifting of position across all three sets of substances—and prescription medicines as well—at the end of the twentieth century and in the first decade of the twenty-first. It also looks at how the factors identified earlier in the book came into play to underpin this process of boundary shift.

Some commentators argued that public health itself was changing as a discourse and practice, away from 'risk' and self-determination which had characterized it in the 1970s and beyond, and towards a focus on precaution. What is clear is that some of the longer-term issues which had served to accelerate the division of the substances from the late nineteenth century through to the mid twentieth were operating to bring them closer together in more recent times. The culture of use was in flux. New sets of professionals and forms of science had entered the substance arena, and public health itself, the 'new' arrival on the post-war scene, was changing to accommodate these new scientific direc-tions. Social movements were influential but in a different way to their operation in the nineteenth century. The dominant technologies now were those of the pharmaceutical industry, and much of the action was conceived at the international and global level.

Drugs for all? Repositioning across licit and illicit drugs

In the last chapter we looked at the reconceptualization of 'public health' so that both in concept and in practice, it moved closer to medi-cine. Medical treatments became public health interventions. This reordering of 'public health' and 'medical' was paralleled by a blurring of the boundaries between recreational drugs, medical treatment, and the use of drugs more generally in society. The boundaries between licit and illicit use were more permeable than before and illicit drugs also repositioned with medical as well as social usage. Drugs such as cannabis and some psychedelic substances were being reconceptual-ized as 'treatments', while prescription and orthodox medicines were being used in a recreational way.

The realignment of cannabis was the most obvious example of this process. Cannabis had a long history as a medicine. It had been used for centuries in Indian and East Asian medicine, and had been introduced into British medical practice by Dr W. B. O'Shaughnessy in the mid nineteenth century, drawing on his experience of its use in India. But it never really secured much of a niche in Western medicine, in part because of its lack of an identified active principle and consequent uncertainty of action. The mistaken belief that Queen Victoria used cannabis in childbirth mentioned earlier, a canard which has been widely and incorrectly repeated, disguised its quite limited appeal in the Victorian period.[290] It was used for sleeplessness, for neuralgia and dysmenorrhoea and in the last quarter of the nineteenth century, its utility in the treatment of insanity was seriously explored—ironic in view of the later argument that cannabis use was a cause of insanity. But later on it fell out of favour even in that area. Cannabis came under the aegis of international drug control in the 1920s (as we have seen in Chapter 7) and the 1961 Single Convention on Narcotic Drugs restricted it even further. Finally, tincture of cannabis left the British Pharmacopeia in the mid 1970s.[291]

The drug was difficult to research, although the Medical Research Council in Britain did fund studies conducted by the pharmacologist Sir William Paton in the 1960s. In 1973, the discovery of the active principle of cannabis, THC, or tetrahydrocannabinol, by Ralph Mechoulam in Israel, began a period of more active research interest, not least on the part of pharmaceutical companies. Research on cannabis also developed in the USA. Pharmaceutical companies began research programmes aimed at developing synthetic compounds which would retain the medical benefits of THC without its psychoactive effects. This separation was not achieved. Only one licensed drug, Nabilone, emerged from all this effort. Later THC itself underwent clinical trials as an anti-emetic and was approved as a prescription medicine with the trade name Marinol. But neither product made much impact.

Research interest continued and resulted in discoveries which helped to revive the medical use. The pharmacologist Leslie Iversen has noted how new animal behaviour models were developed to investigate the properties of the cannabinoids. Major steps forward were the discovery of the CB1 and CB2 receptors followed by a search for CB1 and CB2 selective ligands. This was followed by a search for possible endogenous ligands for the cannabinoid receptors, culminating in the discovery of a family of naturally occurring lipid signalling molecules, the endocannabinoids, with anandamide the first of these.

But the revival of interest in the medical use of the drug, as distinct from this research activity, came from another direction. This came in part from the increase in recreational use of cannabis in the 1980s and 1990s and the growth of self-medication networks. Another impetus was the interest of AIDS activists in alternative medicines and in access via the emergent internet. Reports and ground-level knowledge of the utility of cannabis in dealing with pain and with sickness also emerged in other areas. In Britain, the role of multiple sclerosis (MS) patients stimulated interest on the part of the Multiple Sclerosis Society, which conducted an anonymous survey of its members, revealing the extent of interest. A number of medical organizations began to review the medical uses of the drug. A report from the British Medical Association in 1997 was followed by an enquiry by the House of Lords Science and Technology Committee, published in 1998. As Iversen, who was expert adviser to this Committee, commented, the reports had little immediate impact, but conferred respectability on the idea of cannabis as a medicine. These were followed by an extensive review by the US Institute of Medicine and then by the Royal College of Physicians. All concluded that there was evidence for genuine medical utility but that more research was needed.

The MRC then sponsored a large-scale clinical trial of cannabis in MS which recruited more than six hundred patients and lasted for a year. The results were mixed but there was evidence for some impact on pain and spasticity. Pharmaceutical companies started to become interested and Geoffrey Guy formed a company, GW Pharmaceuticals, to undertake the development of a standardized herbal cannabis extract and a spray delivery system called Sativex. Guy's background in developing herbal medicines and conventional pharmaceuticals gave him experience and licences were provided by the Medicines Control Agency and the Home Office to enable the company to grow a standard crop of cannabis plants and to undertake clinical trials. Clinical data on Sativex persuaded the Canadian government to approve it as a prescription medicine for treating pain in MS patients and the product was then approved in the UK in June 2010.

There were parallel developments in the USA and in parts of Europe. The Canadian government made a medicinal form of herbal cannabis available as the Dutch had done some years earlier. In the USA, voters in several states approved the medical use of smoked cannabis and 'cannabis pharmacies' were set up, although with opposition from the

Federal government. The state of California led this movement and provided state funding for clinical trials. The full use of cannabis products remained to be established—although use of the CB1 antagonist, rimonabant, for the treatment of obesity ended in an expensive failure. Research on cannabis itself and new compounds was largely the province of smaller pharmaceutical or biotechnology companies, but, according to Iversen, writing in 2010, the future looked bright.[292]

Other 'drugs' went through a similar process of repositioning between illicit and medical, although none quite reached the state of development achieved by cannabis. LSD was one example which initially moved from 'medical marvel' to revolutionary street drug. Mescaline, the subject of quasi-medical experimentation in the 1890s provided the raw material for the drug d-lysergic acid diethylamide (LSD) synthesized by the Swiss biochemist Albert Hofmann in 1943. In the 1950s the drug was part of the enthusiasm for new drug treatments in psychiatry, including the advent of anti-psychotics with the discovery of chlorpromazine. Its utility as a treatment for alcoholism was lauded. The desire was to produce an experience which deeply affected the research subjects so that they changed their behaviour; the aim was to restore self-control. In Canada, the widely respected Ontario research agency the Addiction Research Foundation, did its own LSD experiments in the mid 1960s. In the time-honoured way of medical research at that period, many of the leading figures in LSD work also experimented on themselves and on friends and relatives. The rise of what became called 'psychedelic psychiatry' began to encompass a wider philosophical, spiritual, and scientific aspect of drug experimentation. The military began to experiment with LSD as a 'truth drug' and in California, Timothy Leary incorporated psychedelic drug use into a pseudo intellectual movement aimed at developing inner freedoms, supported by LSD advocates such as Ken Kesey. Research declined because of the difficulty of obtaining grants and by the end of the 1960s the drug had definitely been repositioned as unorthodox and 'non-medical'. In the USA the publication of the 1969 LeDain Report on the non-medical use of drugs decisively condemned psychedelic psychiatry, and the UN and WHO came out against it.[293] It seemed that LSD had moved in the opposite direction to cannabis.

But in the early twenty-first century there was a revival of interest in the 'medical' use of the drug and related substances. In 2006 there were experiments with psilocybin at Johns Hopkins medical centre aimed at the treatment of cluster headaches. In England work was stimulated by the Beckley Foundation, a drug policy think tank. It developed a psyche-delic research programme with Imperial College which published results in 2012. This used the vivid images stimulated by use of the drug to propose that it might be a new direction in the treatment of depres-sion.[294] Psychedelics looked possibly set on a boundary change back towards the 'licit' end of the spectrum.

Heroin itself also repositioned both as medicine and as addiction treatment/maintenance drug. It was banned for medical usage in the USA but the British medical profession had successfully resisted attempts by the USA in the 1950s to apply this restriction on a world-wide basis. Heroin (as diacetylmorphine) remained in medical use in the UK for the pain of terminal cancer. It was used by the mass mur-derer GP Dr Harold Shipman in his killing of patients in the 1990s, but the case did not lead to a major reduction in its use. Its use in the treat-ment of addiction underwent a limited international revival from the 1990s. In 1994 the Swiss opened their first heroin maintenance clinics as a three year trial. Late in 1997, the Federal government approved a large expansion of provision, in part motivated to head off the legaliza-tion debate but also as a preventive strategy for HIV/AIDS. The evalu-ation was led by the respected drugs researcher, Ambrose Uchtenhagen, and the results were debated—was the result due to heroin or to better services? Heroin trials were internationally controversial—the Interna-tional Narcotics Control Board (INCB) authorized the importation of heroin and commissioned its own evaluation. This was critical of the research design but in general the trial showed the feasibility of heroin maintenance and improvements in health and social functioning. In a referendum in November 2008, 68 per cent of Swiss voters were in favour of the continuance of heroin maintenance. There were also trials in Germany and the Netherlands; one trial in Australia was aborted. Guidance on heroin prescription published by Britain's National Treatment Agency in 2003 stressed the utility of prescribing the drug as a last resort and under specialist medical control.[295] In 2009, the NAOMI trial reported evidence about heroin prescribing from North America and Europe. Heroin prescription was recognized in some European countries as the optimal treatment for patients for whom options were running out and for whom methadone maintenance had not worked. Heroin prescription kept the user in contact with drug services.[296] This was a far cry from the maintenance image of heroin in the interwar years but it was also a repositioning of the 'drug' as a form of addiction 'medicine'.

This repositioning was a trend across a wider range of substances. What counted as a medicine or a drug was in flux. Back in the 1930s, Aldous Huxley had envisaged a 'brave new world' in which the drug 'soma' would be taken to solve problems or to take a break from harsh reality. This type of use was expanding but also gaining the stamp of official approval. The medical use of cannabis had re-emerged through self-medication by users and the influence of grassroots use was common to the much-changing drug use at the turn of the century. Ecstacy was one such drug. First synthesized in 1914, it had little impact on any market until the chemist, Alexander Shulgin, re-synthesized it and gave it to some therapist friends who used it for their patients. His book PIHKAL (phenoethylamines I have known and loved) went onto the internet and stimulated interest in the increasing number of new synthetic drugs. The mass popularity of Ecstasy began in the 1980s, and was linked to the emergence of the rave scene. But its medical usage was also under investigation and development. Recipes for making Ecstacy and related drugs could be found on the internet.

A whole area of 'legal highs', compounds not controlled under illicit drug regulation because of their changing chemical composition, were also to be found online. Such products were hard to keep up with in terms of control. There was a European 'early warning' system from the late 1990s and risk assessments were made on a European level by the European drug monitoring centre in Lisbon. By 2004 over twenty of the phenethylamines had been brought under control. Tryptamines were less common and some were not active orally. These 'designer drugs' were sometimes called 'legal highs' or 'herbal highs' (herbal seemed safer). They were called chemicals so that medicines legislation did not apply to them. They were ubiquitous and new, uncontrolled, products could be created just be altering a molecule or two.[297] Their availability on the internet highlighted a new drug-focused lifestyle choice. New disorders emerged such as ADD (attention deficit disorder) for which medication was said to be required. A process of medicalization of everyday life was also taking place.

There was a trend for the use of medicines in areas such as the control of mood to become more acceptable. 'We are now starting', said the Foresight leaders in 2007, 'to see the use of cognition enhancers by the healthy.'[298] Drugs developed as medicines were found and used by healthy people. For example, cognition enhancers, drugs which improve mental functioning, sometimes developed to deal with the diseases of the elderly, were being used by healthy people. Methylphenidate (Ritalin) a treatment for ADHD and Modafinil, a treatment for narcolepsy, were being used to improve alertness and performance by groups such as students. What Foresight called 'mental cosmetics' could become accepted and create new expectations about the performance and behaviour of individuals and groups. In 2012 a survey conducted for the *Guardian* newspaper revealed the extent of this boundary-crossing drug use. The paper reported:

> You probably know one or two of Britain's 'hidden' drug users, and may even be one yourself. They are often young, highly educated, working, sociable, and sporty. They feel healthy, happy in their relationships, and confident about the future. They take cannabis, cocaine, MDMA (ecstasy), and, lest we forget, a fair amount of tobacco and alcohol.
>
> It is easy to imagine many of them as smart, respectable, economically productive, holding down jobs in—or preparing to enter—the professions, business, banking, public service, the law, even politics. It's easy to think of these 'happy' drug users as unproblematic: as rational,

self-regulating, middle-class 'consumers' who are relatively discreet and (on the whole), discriminating in their drug use, and who tend to tidy up after themselves.[299]

The twenty-first century in addition saw the British government promoting a 'happiness agenda', a term associated with the LSE economist Lord Layard, which aimed to measure happiness and to survey such feelings in the population. Opponents criticized this on many counts, but it also seemed likely to further 'normalize' pharmaceutical enhancements which helped with happy feelings. 'Wellbeing' was something which policy aimed to enhance.

How did the factors identified earlier in the book promote or underpin these changes? The chapter will now turn to examine some of those earlier issues and how they came to impact in rather different ways in the late twentieth and early twenty-first centuries.

The role of industry and technology now focused on the expanding role of the pharmaceutical industry, both as a more general force in society and as a player in policy development. Critics argued that the industry had too much influence on governments, constantly constructing new illnesses which required expensive new treatments. Diagnosis was now related to the statistical likelihood of developing disease in the future and pathologies such as high blood pressure, diabetes and high cholesterol were only measurable with diagnostic technology. The new epidemiological estimation of risk which accompanied the postwar reorientation of public health also incorporated a new role for the pharmaceutical industry as the provider of medicines which played a key role in the redefinition of chronic disease, as we saw in the previous chapter.[300]

In a more specific way, the industry became connected with new initiatives in tobacco control and in drug treatment. The Robert Woods Johnson Foundation in the USA, based on funding from its initial pharmaceutical industry background, began donating heavily to anti-smoking interests. Glaxo Wellcome, Pfizer, and Pharmacia all became supporters of WHO's tobacco free initiative—these firms were all makers or distributors of drugs such as Nicoderm, Zyban, and Nicorette.

Billions were made by NRT products; in 2007 Nicorette and Nicoderm were selling to the tune of $625 million a year. In 2003 the launch event for WHO's framework convention on tobacco control was funded by the Robert Woods Johnson Foundation, and GlaxoSmith Kline. One aim was to ban nicotine from tobacco—leaving pharmaceutical companies as the main purveyors of the drug.[301] But there were other developments. Tobacco companies were also moving into the nicotine product area. In Sweden the company Niconovum was founded in 2000 to provide clean nicotine products, offering nicotine gum, a nicotine mouth spray and *snus*, Swedish smokeless tobacco. Start up funding was provided by Swedish Match, but in 2009 the company was acquired by R. J. Reynolds the second largest tobacco company in the USA. Tobacco companies were beginning to reposition themselves in the pharmaceutical field.[302]

A similar process was at work in the drugs field, at least in the UK. The focus on methadone and other pharmaceutical interventions as treatment/prevention strategies gave the industry much greater interest in the illicit drug field. When the author attended the National Drug Treatment Conference in 2006, the pharmaceutical industry presence was striking. The conference itself was sponsored by Schering Plough, a company which produced Subutex (Buprenorphine) and Suboxone (Buprenorphine and Naltrexone). A range of other companies with pharmaceutical links and services had stands and had organized breakfast meetings.[303] However, when the author attended another of these conferences in 2009, the pharmaceutical presence was less obvious. More stringent economic times and subsequently the changing treatment agenda of the coalition government, towards 'recovery' and abstinence and away from methadone, may lead to a decline in overt involvement. But the pharmaceutical agenda for drugs was a widening one. Illicit drugs were part of the vaccine development agenda which became such a prominent part of international public health in the twenty-first century. Cocaine vaccines were still several years away in 2012, but there was also research on vaccines to block opiates. Naltrexone implants (NTX) to block the effect of opiates when relapse was highly likely, just after withdrawal, had developed. One implant could block very large doses of opiate for around six months. It remained unlicensed except in Russia where methadone maintenance remained illegal and NTX implants were the only treatment available. In the USA a depot, or longer acting NTX injection, Vivitrol, was licensed for treating opiate dependence. Interest was rising in the UK in line with the government's focus on the 'recovery' agenda. The pharmaceutical route was also more prominent for alcohol than it had been. There was a revival of interest in Disulfiram (DSF, Antabuse) the drug used in the 1940s as a form of aversion therapy for alcoholism. Even the residential rehabilitation centres in the USA, which had been opposed to any form of medication, were beginning to use NTX and also medications for alcoholism.[304] Such trends raised ethical concerns about human rights and consent. The spectre of a mass medicated population loomed large.

What of the role of social movements? The role of voluntary organizations was influential for both tobacco and for illicit drugs. But there were interesting divergences between organizations focused on the different substances and the line they took. Whereas in the nineteenth century the anti-opium movement had been very strongly opposed to the drug's use, the social movement focused on drugs in recent years took a different stance. Drugs networks were very different to the anti-opium international movement of the nineteenth century. They developed a strong focus on harm reduction and 'safe' drug use. The mantle of the nineteenth-century temperance and anti-opium organizations was inherited instead by the anti-tobacco international networks. These anti-tobacco organizations developed a strong abstinence, anti-industry focus. Let us look at those organizations first. We saw this in Chapter 9 with the development of ASH in the UK, which became the model for public health pressure groups and activist organizations more generally. In the 1980s and 1990s what were termed 'advocacy coalitions' became important mechanisms for science-based activism and new players entered the stage. The role of the BMA developed for anti-smoking. The Association was reconstructing its doctor-focused and rather fusty image in the 1980s with greater involvement in social campaigning and public health issues. Smoking became a BMA issue from 1984 and it took a forthright stand against the risk reduction opportunities possible through the chewing tobacco Skoal Bandits, against tobacco advertising, and also charitable investment in tobacco companies. It launched *The Big Kill*, a statistical analysis of smoking related death and disease published in fifteen regional volumes. The BMA set up a Tobacco Alliance which had most of the key players in the field; together they had more publicity than would have been achieved separately. The advent of National No Smoking Day in the early 1980s also led to the cancer charities becoming involved. The activities of this anti-smoking coalition were described in a BMA report *Smoking Out the Barons* published in 1986. This advocacy coalition also developed at the European and international levels during the 1980s.

Networks had first developed in the 1970s. The World Conferences on smoking and health became an important meeting place for smoking researchers and activists. The first was held in New York in 1967, with Robert Kennedy as keynote speaker, followed by one in London in 1971. George Godber, the former Chief Medical Officer (CMO), who had been instrumental in pushing forward the first Royal College of Physicians report on smoking in 1962, gave a rousing address, 'It Can be Done'. He looked to international networks to take forward the anti-smoking case. Older international organizations changed to take on tobacco as an issue. Sir John Crofton in Edinburgh, and his wife Eileen, were early advocates of smoking control through his initial interest in tuberculosis (TB). In his unpublished autobiography, he recalled how the International Union against Tuberculosis (IUAT) became the International Union against TB and Lung Disease (IUATLD) in 1984. It set up a special committee on smoking. Crofton and Kjell Bjartveit from Norway produced a booklet, *The Smoking Epidemic: How You Can Help* which was distributed to all IUATLD members and affiliated organizations.

The role of personalities was important and also the cross-national transfer of national experiences. A key figure was Nigel Gray in Australia, director of the Anti-Cancer Council of Victoria from 1968 until 1995. Gray became the Director of the smoking work of the International Union against Cancer in 1974. Here was another international organization which, with Norwegian funding, changed its emphasis and began to do work in developing countries. Successful examples of anti-tobacco activity were used as models for action internationally. Gray's work on the Victoria Anti-Tobacco Act of 1987 which raised taxes and restricted advertising was used in this way.

The pace quickened. More organizations were developing an international focus—for example David Simpson, the Director of British ASH, set up his International Agency on Tobacco and Health, which specifically focused on low-income countries and on Eastern Europe. It focused on information dissemination, on providing the tools for activism.

Europe started to play a role—the impetus came with the establishment in 1987 of the Europe against Cancer programme, initially as a response to Chernobyl, but also expanding its remit as Europe developed its competence to take on matters of public health. Directives and resolutions on tobacco began to be adopted there in the late 1980s and early 1990s. Between 1989 and 1992 seven directives and one non-binding resolution on tobacco were adopted.[305] The role of developing countries also became important and with this a realization that tobacco was an international trade and tobacco industries were transnational. Regional action plans were set up and groups of public health researchers coalesced round the tobacco issue. One leading health economist, Joy Townsend, spoke of how the health economists who worked on smoking became like a brotherhood.

> There developed very strong international tobacco control community which is still growing fast. It is like a brotherhood with a strong commitment to sharing evidence, data and policy ideas. It consists of members of NGOs, UICC, WHO, Union against TB and Lung disease, smoke free partnerships, ASH, CRUK, Tobacco Free Kids and many, many more.[306]

Alcohol was part of this process of social movement formation. It likewise developed an alliance founded on public health and psychiatric interests. Some commentators referred to a neo-temperance alliance around alcohol dating from the coalition of organizations which had produced the 'purple book' in the 1970s. Of course this was very different from temperance in that it was a coalition of researchers with no grass roots organization. This coalition continued to frame the terms of the public health debate into the early twenty-first century through publications such as *Alcohol Policy and the Public Good* (1994) and *Alcohol: No Ordinary Commodity* (2003). The coalition, like that for tobacco, took a strongly anti-industry line and promoted a 'whole population' approach for alcohol—that government intervention should be through taxation (later modified to minimum pricing, another economic lever) and control of advertising. This health coalition lost momentum however in the early twenty-first century in the UK in the face of a strong public order lobby based on the police, focusing on public disorder and the regulation of the 'night-time economy'. The health lobby subsequently re-formed—away from psychiatry—with liver specialists and those working in hospital Accident and Emergency departments playing a lead role. The leader of the new Alcohol Alliance in the UK was Sir Ian Gilmore, a liver specialist and former president of the Royal College of Physicians. The public debate was around cirrhosis deaths and liver disease rather than alcohol problems and alcoholism. But the 'alcohol movement' sought to learn from tobacco and the ways in which that 'drug' had been detached from mainstream culture over a fifty year period.

The biggest change was in social movement involvement in the drugs issue. Whereas the nineteenth-century anti-opium movement had strongly opposed the non-medical use of opium in the Far East, and taken a prohibitionist stance, in the late twentieth and early twenty-first centuries a very different type of national and international movement grew up, which focused on post-AIDS harm reduction. The history of drug voluntarism and radicalism can be tracked before the 1980s through organizations in the UK such as Release, or the therapeutic communities, or the Community Drugs project.[307] The role of the drug addict as 'user' or consumer of drugs had became more central and AIDS accelerated this trend. Legalization of drugs had never attracted mainstream support but harm reduction as a cause had a different ethos and could attract a broader coalition of interests. The International Harm Reduction Association (IHRA) established initially in Liverpool in the 1980s developed into an international coalition which lobbied for harm reduction policies. A coalition of these types of organization, civil society organizations, was in operation by the 2010s, funded by the Beckley Foundation and advocating harm reduction and human rights for drug users. A group of Nordic drug researchers characterized the change which had taken place. Whereas groups in the national context often appeared 'weak, fragmented and marginalized…the picture is very different if we look at them not as separate and isolated national phenomena, but rather as part of a broader transnational current'. They argued:

> The idea of a movement becomes more relevant when the minor associations are considered as part of a more widespread trend that seeks to address, question and even challenge the conditions and policies that define and structure drug users' lives.[308]

So the positioning of social movements served also to bring the substances into a closer relationship. The tobacco social movement argued for greater restrictions on the substance, a generally more restrictive attitude, while the drug coalitions in general wanted drugs to be regulated but in such a way that harm to their users was reduced. The greater restriction for tobacco and the lessening restriction for drugs, again was a trend which brought the substances closer.

And increasingly such arguments were made and activities took place at the international or global level. Internationalism or international control, was an important motive force, as it had also been historically. The international drugs networks and coalitions were trying to secure modification of the international drug control treaties, while the tobacco networks sought to secure international action primarily through the promulgation, under the aegis of WHO, of an international framework convention on tobacco. The international drug control machinery, which we left in Chapter 7 in the interwar period, had then primarily been a system of control of supply with strong influence from the colonial nations with an interest in opium. But during and after the Second World War, it had come under the strong and prohibitionist influence of the United States and the personality of the US drug 'czar' Harry Anslinger. The USA had worked to secure a more restrictionist approach including the ending of the opium monopolies in countries such as India. As the historian John Collins has shown, such a punitive approach was by no means predetermined but it did set the tone of postwar international drug control. The Americans also showed themselves willing to ally drug control with their political agendas overseas, as had been the case since the days of the Shanghai Commission.[309]

In the drugs field by the 1990s, there was an ongoing lobby to secure more harm reduction measures through the United Nations machinery and the Commission on Narcotic Drugs (CND). Activists from IHRA, Human Rights Watch, the Canadian HIV AIDS Legal Network, the Beckley Foundation, and the Open Society Institute tried to gain access to CND meetings. Cracks were appearing in the international drug control system and countries which had signed decades before were seeking ways in which they could modify the more draconian provisions. In the early twenty-first century, these moves went further, with a Latin American Commission in 2007 on drugs and democracy and the 2011 Global Commission on Drugs Policy, which saw a host of high-profile world leaders call for decriminalization. The president of Columbia spoke in favour of the decriminalization of cannabis.

The best option seemed to be for countries to reassert the possibility of adopting a system of regulation within national boundaries while meeting obligations under the treaty to control the international trade in drugs. So a country could withdraw from one or more of the treaties and then re-accede with specified reservations. Bolivia, for example, wished to recognize the cultural use of the coca leaf and so planned to renounce the treaty and then to re-sign with an addendum. This could develop as a more general model for change at the international level.

Meanwhile, the International Narcotics Control Board maintained a hard-line stance, with criticism of countries such as Afghanistan which were in breach of their obligations under the treaty. Civil society organizations pointed to what appeared to be double standards, in that the Board was not critical of Thailand which imposed the death penalty for drugs offences. The medical use of cannabis appeared to offer a particular challenge to international control and there was discussion of a possible framework convention for that drug on the lines of tobacco. In 2012, leading researchers Robin Room and Peter Reuter gave a summing up which encapsulated that state of flux at the national and international levels and the shifting boundaries around drug definition.

> The cultural positions of different drugs vary enough to preclude universal policies on how to deal with all illicit or indeed licit drugs. From the perspective of public health, we need to move towards a control system that is more aligned with the risks that different drugs pose to users.[310]

Such activities were aimed at modifying control mechanisms.

Meanwhile, in the tobacco field, activists aimed a greater, not lessening control, although not on the drugs model. The international networks began to press WHO for action, leading ultimately to international control of tobacco in the early twenty-first century. Tobacco belatedly adopted the international regulation model. Progress within WHO was initially slow. There was only one officer in Geneva in the 1980s, Roberto Masironi, with a small budget and little support. Crofton, and John Reid, CMO for Scotland, who was also on the WHO Board, met Halfdan Mahler, Director General (DG) of WHO, and tried to persuade him to take up the issue. Despite a couple of reports from expert committees, the issue had not been very prominent and Mahler agreed, at the 6th international conference in Tokyo in 1987, to convene a group to prepare a Global Action Plan on Tobacco and Health. This met in Geneva in 1988 with Judith McKay as rapporteur. Although adopted by the World Health Assembly unanimously in 1988, matters stalled again with the advent of Nakajima as DG and changes in the tobacco unit which caused some disruption.

Personalities and new areas of research were crucial. The role of one doctor, Judith McKay, was important. McKay had been a student of the Croftons in Edinburgh in the 1960s and attributed her subsequent interest in smoking to their influence. China became an area of concern, in part because of her work. Changes in epidemiological research also impacted. Richard Peto's epidemiological research went global, looking at the implications of the 'smoking epidemic' for China. Murray and Lopez in their *World Development Report* in 1993 highlighted tobacco and Lopez moved into WHO tobacco control.

Hirayama's research on passive smoking emanated from Japan. New forms of epidemiology were based on new international networks. In the crucial area of health economics, similar networks developed. The health economist Joy Townsend recalled how she first became involved at a World Conference in Winnipeg in 1983 and how subsequently a very strong international tobacco control constituency developed within health economics. The World Bank became involved and its report *Curbing the Epidemic*, was published in 1999.

Matters came to a head in the 1990s. There was pressure from without. In 1993, Ruth Roemer at UCLA, with long standing WHO advisory connections, and Allyn Taylor decided to apply to tobacco control Taylor's argument that WHO had the constitutional power to develop international conventions to advance global health. Despite initial opposition by WHO officials, the idea gained wide acceptance for tobacco. A head of steam from outside was important. Roemer brought the issue to the first All-Africa conference on Tobacco or Health co-chaired by Derek Yach, who was then with the Medical Research Council (MRC) of South Africa. Strong support emerged from Judith McKay, by then director of the Asian consultancy for tobacco control, who helped with drafting a resolution at the 9th World Conference in Paris in 1994.

Support came from Jean Lariviere, a senior medical adviser at Health Canada, who drafted a resolution tabled at the WHO executive board in January 1995. It requested that the DG report to the Board on the feasibility of developing an international convention.

McKay was a key figure in pushing this forward and in promoting the idea of a framework convention rather than a code, as had been the case with breast milk substitutes. The election of Gro Harlem Brundtland as DG in 1998 made a difference. Matters had developed so far but there was still a lack of support at the political and global level. Her two priorities were tobacco control and malaria. A Tobacco Free Initiative, headed by Yach, was charged with developing the framework convention. Brundtland had been the Norwegian Prime Minister and had experience within WHO and the UN—she had been commissioner of the sustainable development commission for the Secretary General in the 1980s and knew how to get things done.

The growth and influence of coalitions was important, encompassing both rich and poor countries and those in between. The example of how such coalitions had operated to mobilize support for other areas, such as in the environmental field, was drawn upon. Canada had a long track record in international public health, dating back to the Lalonde report in the 1970s. But resource-poor countries and countries like Brazil, one of the top three tobacco growing countries, were also involved. France, Finland, and Switzerland made contributions to get the treaty underway. NGOs from the south also helped drive the process. South Africa and Kenya were centrally involved. The other UN agencies were brought on board with a Secretary General's task force on tobacco control operating from 1999.

Even the industry could see some advantages to the new system. Philip Morris and the Big Three realized that it might be an opportunity for them. It would open markets, give them more power, destroy smaller companies, and make the bigger ones grow. The convention split the industry. A country such as Japan with a strong national tobacco industry worked in the opposite direction, to water down the convention. The ongoing revelations of tobacco industry archives from the late 1990s also put pressure on and aided activism; so a form of history had its role to play.

In 1996 the WHO voted to proceed with development of the convention, it was adopted in 2003 and came into force in 2005. There have been further networks developing since then. The treaty strengthened the international tobacco NGO community. The Framework Convention Alliance was set up in 1999 and is made up of over thirty-five organizations from 100 countries working on the development of the treaty. Funding from the Bloomberg initiative and from Gates has followed, offering serious financial support for tobacco control in low and middle income countries.[311] The framework convention was consciously set up as a different model from international drug control. In the early twenty-first century, there were moves to establish a similar mechanism for alcohol at the international level.

The picture which emerges from the sketch of influences above is of tobacco being repositioned to be more like an illicit drug; while other forms of drug use (legal highs, prescription drugs, cognition enhancers) became more acceptable within society, part of a continuum of drug use and altering consciousness. So the detachment of tobacco from cultural acceptability and repositioning as a 'drug' and 'addictive' was broadly paralleled by a greater acceptability for other forms of drug use. The rise of hedonism and of consumer culture encompassed the use of drugs more than it has that of tobacco. The emergent role for tobacco as an 'underground' substance was reinforced by the growth of tobacco smuggling, defined as the large scale import and export of tobacco on which no duty has been paid. Smuggling, so public health experts pointed out, was more prevalent in Southern and Eastern European countries where cheap cigarettes predominated, than where prices were much higher.[312] 'Smuggling', they asserted 'appears...to be associated with the presence of organized crime, a culture of street selling, and complicity of the industry'. The fact of smuggling also underlined the changing status and positioning of tobacco.

Fear—and the role of women

Alcohol might seem to be the exception to this repositioning of the substances and realignment of the boundaries between them. It seemed at first sight to retain its position as a culturally accepted, even encouraged substance. But there were signs of change. If we turn to a further issue considered previously, that of fear, we can see that a process of 'deculturing' of alcohol was beginning to get under way, although how far it would reach was open to speculation. Alcohol re-emerged as a policy issue in a number of countries in the 1990s and early twenty-first century; the UK (or rather England, as devolved Scotland was distinctively different) will be used as the example here. Fear of alcohol use was bound up with that traditional issue of womens' drinking and also with public order issues. The Labour government had actively promoted the 'night-time economy', in particular through the 2003 Licensing Act which allowed 24-hour drinking. This was accompanied by a number of changes which fuelled concern—among them a focus in research on high-risk drinkers rather than simply risky drinking; a change in the government's policy on alcohol units which cited daily unit intake rather than overall weekly unit consumption (and thus encouraged a focus on daily drink intake). Concern about disorder in city centres was initially led by the police rather than by medical interests and in some cases emanated from police concerns about declining funding and support.[313]

As was traditional, fear of alcohol use was expressed through the role of women. Binge drinking became a preoccupation of journalists and politicians with a dramatic rise in the use of the terminology after 2004. *The Times* began to use the term in the late 1990s, with between ten and twenty mentions a year between 1998 and 2002, then a doubling for the year 2003 (thirty-nine mentions). However, 2004 saw a three-fold increase in the number of articles including the term 'binge drinking'. Many of these articles were related to the changes to licensing laws enshrined in the Licensing Act 2003. Here are a just a few of the headlines:

Blitz on binge drinking to curb violence (*The Times*, 29 April 2004).
Just one more binge for the road (an article about high earning women and drinking, *The Times* 27 May 2005).
Drink laws will cause teen deaths warns liver doctor (*The Times*, 29 August 2005)
Drinking blamed for big rise in violence (*The Times*, 29 October 2005)

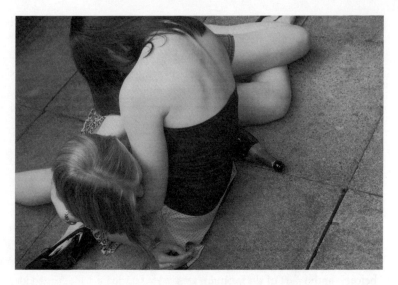

FIGURE 10 Binge drinking women.

Researchers pointed out that the definition of what binge drinking actually was was confused; that the proportion of men 'binge drinking' was much higher than women; and that levels of drinking were actually beginning to go down.[314] But this carried little weight against a frenzy of media interest which was determined to seek out party-going female twenty-somethings in city centres with short skirts and 'attitude'. A German TV crew interviewing the author in c. 2005 about binge drinking was determined, despite evidence that men should be their target, to seek out some good shots of drunken women—it went down so much better with the viewers.[315]

Alcohol in this way seemed to be beginning the process of cultural change which had affected tobacco twenty to thirty years before, when passive smoking first came on to the scene. In fact, alcohol activists consciously discussed what might be the 'passive smoking' tactic to use for alcohol. 'Harm to others' became the mantra in the alcohol field and researchers began to gather together and to quantify how this might be calculated. A key statistic would have more impact than other modes of discussion. What did emerge by way of the 'harm to others'/'innocent victim' style of argument again focused on women and children. It was encapsulated in the issue of foetal alcohol syndrome (FAS) and women's drinking during pregnancy. Two US researchers, Armstrong and Abel, one of whom had spent part of his working life working in the area of FAS, drew attention to the 'discovery' of FAS in the early 1970s in the USA at a time of concern about alcohol more generally in society and an increase in child abuse. As with the concept of addiction and inebriety in the late nineteenth century, wider social and cultural forces gave the concept significance. Armstrong and Abel pointed out that concerns and responses had escalated by the end of the century way beyond what the evidence supported. American style 'new abstinence' movements such as Mothers Against Drunk Driving (MADD) and biomedical researchers united round a position where any drinking during pregnancy or even before, on the part of the woman, was risky and to be condemned as a form of 'child abuse'. The Surgeon General's guidelines on drinking in pregnancy mandated abstinence with no exceptions.

In Britain, a different attitude initially prevailed. The Royal College of Obstetricians and Gynaecologists 1996 guidelines saw no harm in drinking up to a unit of alcohol a day during pregnancy; this was also the more general European response to the issue. But in the twenty-first century official advice changed. In 2007, the Department of Health issued new guidelines which stressed not only that pregnant women should not drink at all but that anyone trying to get pregnant should also cease using alcohol. The new guidelines were not uncontroversial, in particular since they recognized that there was no new evidence to support this recommendation.[316] Researchers in the field had concluded that FAS was a rare outcome of drinking in pregnancy and indeed was not always connected with drinking at all. However, the focus on poorer drinking women was typical of the deculturing process which had also affected tobacco earlier on—through the image of the smoking pregnant mother. The rise of the new abstinence model for alcohol and women was also apparent in other European countries, for example in Denmark and Finland, which also modified their advice to pregnant women, despite a lack of evidence.[317] The Australian national guidelines also recommended no drinking in pregnancy. In the UK this marked one area of rapprochement between the alcohol industry and campaigning interests. The drinks industry funded advice to pregnant women not to drink. It was significant that fear of women was one area which united these usually opposed interests.

Harsher attitudes were developing for female and also for lower-class consumers of alcohol in general. The traditional boundary between health and criminal justice concerns which had marked the initial development of the 'inebriety' model in the late nineteenth century had been redefined in the twenty-first century through the development of initiatives such as drug and drink treatment and testing orders. Part of a broader law and order agenda associated with the Labour government, which included anti-social behaviour orders (ASBOs), the more recent possibilities included 'tagging' of offenders to make sure that they did not drink. One Justice of the Peace involved with the process commented that they were clearly stigmatizing lower-class poorer drinkers who came to the attention of the courts, not the middle-class drinkers whose consumption was also problematic.[318] The focus was on women and the lower classes, not 'us': alcohol consumption was becoming aligned with the 'other'.

The impact on regulation

What impact had all this in terms of actual regulation? In later years, regulation was also in flux, although little of this filtered into public discussion. We will look at the trend to reposition drugs and tobacco in particular.

The issue of public space and its regulation highlighted the role of fear and its application across the substances. In Britain, government regulation allowed local byelaws instituting alcohol-free public spaces, alongside those which were drug free. A similar control of space came for smoking in Britain in 2005 when a total smoking ban was introduced in all public places. Although the Labour government had published the first ever White Paper on tobacco in 1998, it had continued a voluntary approach to controlling smoking in public places. By the early 2000s, there was pressure within government to move to a statutory ban; the Labour Party's 2005 manifesto proposed only a partial one. But the full ban came about through a series of complex manoeuvres. At a 'policy reunion' of some of the key players, it was generally agreed that the move to a total ban illustrated the power of parliament and in particular of its select committee process.[319] The comprehensive ban went with the grain of public opinion, and it also had vocal support from the Chief Medical Officer, Sir Liam Donaldson, representative of the public health community. The willingness of powerful Health Secretaries (John Reid and Patricia Hewitt) to argue for action; and the tactical use of the Health Select Committee under a committed chair, the Labour MP Kevin Barron, were also important. The Committee's visit to Ireland, which had already instituted a ban, and to a pub in Killarney, was a media-hyped event. But a crucial turning point came when the hospitality trade shifted its position to support a total ban. The industry was concerned to maintain a 'level playing field' in the industry in terms of the measures to be adopted and eventually it unified round the total approach. The tobacco industry failed to build any sort of effective alliance to oppose it. Evidence that was gathered after the ban had been in place for a few years cast doubt on its effectiveness in reducing smoking rates. But its symbolic significance was great. It marked a continuing detachment of tobacco from mainstream culture and also a realignment with both alcohol and drugs in terms of the regulation of visibility and of public space. Further discussion of plain packaging for cigarettes and the removal of cigarettes from open sale in 2012 reinforced this trend.

The public debate was still around legalization as opposed to the 'war on drugs'; or, in the case of tobacco, the need for more stringent controls on availability and use. But there had been interesting attempts to change forms of regulation in the past for tobacco and also other more recent initiatives for drugs. For tobacco, the moves had tried to bring the substance under different structures of regulation. In the 1970s in Britain, the then Health Minister, David Owen, had tried to bring tobacco substitutes, which were being developed, under the provisions of the 1968 Medicines Act, so that they would be controlled like medicines. The idea was that tobacco itself would eventually go down the same route. Owen operated cleverly, using ASH adroitly and leaking information to sections of the industry who were sympathetic. The British-based Imperial Tobacco, long an ally of government, was 'on side', while the USA owned sections of the industry (Rothmans, Gallahers, Phillip Morris, and BAT) were not. Owen astutely recognized that the most significant section of the British industry—Imperial—had interests potentially overlapping with those of the government and of its independent committee of scientists. In an interview with a journalist in 1976 he commented:

> Now what they have is a commercial interest which wants them to go down the Medicines Act. Because they know that we will not dare give them permission for additives and substitutes under the present provision…Those who want to go into the substitutes and additives market, which Imperial strongly wants to do, they can see that once this mechanism is going, first of all they get some sort of security from being given a licence…I have always made it absolutely clear to them that I was prepared to do a section 105 order on a compromise basis, but that if they forced me into the position of going to substantive legislation in the next session…I would not dream of doing a partial thing…it can be a very short bill to put tobacco under the Medicines Act.[320]

These initiatives eventually came to nothing because of the failure of substitutes and Owen's move from Health to the Foreign Office in 1976.

The realignment of tobacco as a medicine or pharmaceutical re-emerged as an issue in the 1990s when there were US moves to regulate nicotine-containing tobacco products as medical devices under the aegis of the Food and Drug Administration (FDA). In 1996, David Kessler, head of the FDA, announced that the agency would regulate nicotine-containing tobacco products as medical devices, restrict youth access to tobacco products, and restrict tobacco advertising that might appeal to children.

In 1984, the Food, Drugs, and Cosmetic Act (FDA) had approved Nicorette chewing gum used as 'replacement therapy', so Kessler was regulating these products but had no jurisdiction over the product they sought to replace. But this initiative came to an end when in 2000 the Supreme Court decided against FDA jurisdiction. Tobacco activists then tried to get legislation passed allowing the FDA to regulate tobacco as a drug. Some opposed this tactic because it would make the cigarette 'respectable'. In 2009, the arrival of the Obama Administration saw Congress pass the Family Smoking Prevention and Tobacco Control Act. This added a new chapter to the Federal Food Drug and Cosmetic Act confirming the FDA's authority to regulate tobacco, and thus bypassed the Supreme Court's 2000 decision. A new Centre for Tobacco Products was set up in the FDA, which required the submission of data and research documents on tobacco products, new labelling on cigarettes and smokeless tobacco products (such as chewing tobacco) and new restrictions on advertising and promotion. The administration was authorized to review all new tobacco products to assess whether permitting them to be marketed would be appropriate for the protection of public health. This tactic evolved from the pre-review of pharmaceuticals.[321]

In Britain, the emergence of NRT as a regulated medicine was the inheritor of the 1970s moves round tobacco. There were divergences between the British and American stance on regulation—the UK one aimed to make it available as a therapy while in the USA nicotine was to be more stringently regulated, with a view to elimination. But in both countries, systems of pharmaceutical review were put in place by the early twenty-first century. The EU also decided to regulate electronic cigarettes as medicines in 2013.

Systems of illicit drug regulation were also in flux. The greatest fluidity in systems of illicit drug regulation came in Europe, which had emerged as a 'player' on the substance scene since the 1980s. A European Monitoring Centre on Drugs and Drug Addiction was set up in

1993 and served as a harmonizing influence, especially for research and drug epidemiology, across countries. The Netherlands with its cannabis coffee shops and visible drug use in Amsterdam for a while became a Mecca for those interested in writing about different possibilities for drug regulation. The Dutch policy was actually one of non-enforcement even though cannabis was illegal. The system had evolved from a depenalization regime from the mid 1970s to the mid 1980s, to de facto legalization from the mid 1980s. The latter was distinguished by the commercialization of cannabis through a network of coffee shops engaged in increasingly overt promotion. American researchers Rob MacCoun and Peter Reuter of the Rand Corporation evaluated the effects of depenalization and found that it had no effect on cannabis use. But data from the second decade of liberalization suggested that the commercialization of cannabis was associated with rising levels of use.[322] Such evaluation studies were rare, although generally it was accepted that types of policy did not determine levels of use in societies. There was little link between law enforcement and the prevalence of drug use.

Perhaps with this in mind, a number of European countries embarked on less restrictive regimes for drug control in the late twentieth century. One widely cited example was that of Portugal, where in 2001 possession of a small amount of any drug was made subject to non-criminal penalties or diversion to treatment or education programmes, decided by a non-judicial three-person panel. The outcomes appeared to be good. There were small increases in illicit drug use among adults but reduced illicit drug use among problematic drug users and adolescents detected from 2003, and a reduction in opioid related deaths and infectious diseases. As researchers pointed out, many other factors had also changed over this period, so the impact of legal changes could not be isolated independently.[323]

Drug regimes like those for tobacco/nicotine were in flux in the early twenty-first century and in some European countries the move was towards more 'liberal' modes of control, or pragmatic controls through the use of civil penalties rather than criminalization. In the Netherlands, local political change and pressure from the Schengen partners worried about 'drug tourism' brought greater restriction. Cannabis sales in coffee shops were restricted to local consumers over eighteen and in the possession of a 'ration card', a system with some similarities to the historical Gothenburg one, or even to proposals put forward to a select committee on pharmacy in the UK in the 1850s.

In Britain, too, despite the much publicized change for cannabis from class B to C and back again, the use of civil penalties for drug offences was rising. Community sentences for drug offences had quadrupled in the UK since the mid 1990s and were given to a quarter of drug offenders coming before the courts in 2010. Starting with Drug Treatment and Testing Orders in 2000 the criminal justice system was also being used to get users into treatment.[324] Overall too drug use was in decline.

Khat and the process of transition

The process of transition could also work the other way. Khat, a drug which had a long history as a stimulant in Yemen and Ethiopia, and later in Kenya, Somalia, and Uganda, became a transnational and international commodity in the late twentieth century through the pressure of migration and displacement. Initially the drug fell under the drug control radar because of the lack of an alkaloid-based 'medicine/drug', its rapid loss of potency, the need for daily flights to import the drug and its confinement to immigrant populations. Khat chewing did not appeal to the hedonist 'happy' drug-taking urban milieu identified in the 2012 *Guardian* survey. But very different views were held at the community level about the substance. Commentators argued about the dangers of criminalizing the use of khat and a high proportion of the Somali population. But Somali women formed a vocal opposition to the use of the drug on the basis of its impact on family life and the ability to work. When the author attended an open session of the ACMD in 2010, grass roots groups opposing khat dominated the public session. Initially the Advisory Council on the Misuse of Drugs reacted in a measured way to pressure for greater controls. In 2005 it concluded

'Khat is a much less potent stimulant than other commonly used drugs such as amphetamine and cocaine. However some individuals use it in a dependent manner.'[325] But the international dimension loomed ever larger. The USA, Canada, and Sweden had criminalized the drug and the transit through Heathrow airport of continuing supplies of the drug caused concern. The ACMD came under international pressure to review the situation. Researchers who had looked at khat predicted what the future might hold if criminalization proceeded.

In the UK, the khat trade has provided fledgling Somali entrepreneurs with a business opportunity where they can operate with advantage and accumulate capital. There is no reported diversificiation into other drugs, and the police emphatically dissociate khat use and distribution from organized crime...When supply is cut while demand remains high the market will reconfigure underground. Business transactions will assume all the features of a criminal drug economy, and the supply

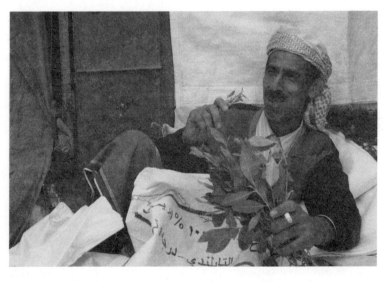

FIGURE 11 Khat chewing. Man enjoying his qat in Sana'a, Yemen, January 2009.

will be taken over by criminals who will eventually consolidate into networks.[326]

The ACMD's review of khat, published in 2013, held the line on further criminalization, although the Home Secretary, Theresa May, decided to reject this advice. The case of khat shows again how economics, social movements, and the international dimension could combine to alter the status of a substance. Like, alcohol, illicit drugs, and tobacco, its status was in flux in the early twenty-first century.

12
Afterword: History and the Future

'Do you believe in the legalization of drugs? I did a programme on the subject', said the TV man as we talked during a medical humanities conference. I stuttered an unconvincing reply, wrong-footed at being asked to declare a position in a debate which I thought missed the point and where his meaning was unclear. Saying 'I wouldn't have started from there' was unlikely to have prolonged the conversation. The argument put forward in this book would have taken more than the coffee break to explain. Nor was it easy to propose that a historian's job was to observe and to analyse change—what had happened and why—rather than to advocate particular courses of action in the future.

Nevertheless what the future might bring is intriguing. The focus of public discussion remains, despite the rise of interest in alcohol in the last few years, on illicit drugs. Popular books on drugs proliferate and fascinate the media.[327,328, 329,330] It is rare for the discussion to encompass a wider range of substances. Prohibition and legalization as banner headlines fulfil useful functions for politicians and the media. Yet the balance of forces across the substances has been shifting, including the way we conceptualize and respond to them. The argument in this book has focused on forces and issues which have brought change in both the 'deeper' and more recent past. The substances now seem to be drawing closer together. In the USA the research organizations for alcohol (NIAAA) and for drugs (NIDA) have merged. The Rand corporation was running sessions in early 2013 looking at public health regulations for marijuana in the light of tobacco and alcohol control. The report of the UK Drug Policy Commission, published in the autumn of 2012, added to the pressure for civil penalties for drug offences, bringing them ever closer to penalties for alcohol and for smoking tobacco. When the UK Drug Policy Commission published the report, the coalition government's rejection of its call for a Royal Commission was widely publicized. The same government's initiation early in 2013 of an enquiry into alternative regulatory regimes such as that in Portugal attracted less attention but was no less significant. Such willingness to examine alternative regimes would not have been possible even a few years earlier.

But it would be unwise to predict the future. There are countervailing forces both nationally and internationally. Control rather than hedonism may be the unifying rhetoric and practice across the substances in the future. The advent, for example, of the 'recovery' agenda in recent UK drug policy could presage greater control over drug use in one segment of the illicit market, a more restrictive approach. Neuroscience, the hope in the USA for a treatment-focused 'disease' agenda, has reinforced the supply side approach and the idea of the 'hijacked brain' has been appropriated by drug warriors and anti-terrorist forces. The introduction of plain packaging for tobacco has connotations of the illicit drug; and tagging alcohol offenders does not fit with the 'happiness' agenda. Criminal justice rather than 'drugs for all' could be the unifying rhetoric. Alcohol consumption, like that of drugs, is currently in decline. Office of National Statistics (ONS) figures showed in 2013 that the trend had been apparent since 2007. Anti-alcohol campaigners sought to derive 'lessons from history', the history in this case being that of anti-tobacco activism with its resolute anti-industry stance. There were in fact many other lessons which could be learnt from the history of tobacco and its 'deculturing'. They were less palatable to campaigners who could not envisage the utility of any alliance with industrial interests. That such a stance had become the norm illustrated a harsher response. This could dovetail with habits which are becoming less prominent in society and where culture is now less consumption focused and more concerned with abstinence. Such a response would at one and the same time further speed the process of control.

But it can safely be predicted that the forces which drive change will include those identified in the preceding chapters. Fear, in particular involving women or the impact on young people and babies, the future of the race, remains as strong, and unthinking, an engine of policy development in the early twenty-first century as it was in the 1900s. A debate in 2012 about offering long-term contraception to drug using women had echoes of eugenics.[331] The role of different national systems remains important but also their positioning in international regulation. Russia, where drug control remains immune from the trends towards harm reduction and patterns of alcohol consumption are much higher than those in Western European societies, has also introduced tobacco control. It is a new prohibitionist power in the system, a potential successor to the USA whose role may be in decline. Internationalism and the role of control, or its absence at the supra national level, affects all countries. There are currently, as discussed in Chapter 11, signs of change within international drug control. Debate currently centres on what might bring further change. An historian would draw attention to the factors which have brought change and movement in the past. Here one can itemize the impact of war; of power politics and agendas larger than drug control; bureaucratic policymaking; and industrial interests, in particular those of the pharmaceutical industry. The role of non-European countries has also been a significant motive force in the history. The colonial interests which were implicated in control, both pro and anti, of the early twentieth century have been replaced by the Latin American countries, which have taken up the issue in the present. Change might be possible given a suitable conjuncture of these forces. And in some respects the different models used for drug control and tobacco control are drawing closer together, with recent calls for a framework convention for cannabis on the model of the one for tobacco.[332]

Whatever the future holds, there will be a need to look behind the immediate headline and to analyse the longer-term processes at work. A re-ordering of substances is indeed possible but the new positioning will be time dependent, the plaything of other issues, not a 'rational' process.

NOTES

CHAPTER 1: INTRODUCTION: PAST AND PRESENT

1. D. Nutt, L. A. King, W. Saulsbury, C. Blakemore, 'Development of a rational scale to assess the harm of drugs of potential misuse', *Lancet*, 369 (2007), 1047–53.
2. M. Gladwell, *The Tipping Point. How Little Things Can Make a Big Difference* (London: Abacus, 2001).
3. T. Seddon, *A History of Drugs. Drugs and Freedom in the Liberal Age* (Abingdon: Routledge/Glass House, 2010), 13.
4. J. Burnett, *Liquid Pleasures. A Social History of Drinks in Modern Britain* (London: Routledge, 1999), 112.
5. Burnett, *Liquid Pleasures*, 142.
6. J. Nicholls, *The Politics of Alcohol. A History of the Drink Question in England* (Manchester: Manchester University Press, 2009), 31, 35–9.
7. J. Goodman, 'Excitantia. Or, how Enlightenment Europe took to soft drugs' in J. Goodman, P. E. Lovejoy, and A. Sherratt, eds. *Consuming Habits. Global and Historical Perspectives on How Cultures Define Drugs* (Abingdon: Routledge, 2007), 2nd edn, 123.
8. J. Goodman, *Tobacco in History. The Cultures of Dependence* (London: Routledge, 1993), 59.
9. Quoted in V. Berridge, *Opium and the People. Opiate Use and Drug Control Policy in Nineteenth and Early Twentieth-Century England* (London: Free Association Books, 1999) expanded edn, xxiii
10. Berridge, *Opium and the People*, 210.
11. Berridge, *Opium and the People*, 216.
12. A. W. Crosby, Jr, *The Columbian Exchange. Biological and Cultural Consequences of 1492* (Westport, CT: Greenwood Publishing Co., 1972).
13. D. Courtwright, *Forces of Habit. Drugs and the Making of the Modern World* (Cambridge, MA: Harvard University Press, 2001), 9.
14. C. Nathanson, 'Social movements as catalysts for policy change: The case of smoking and guns', *Journal of Health Policy, Politics and Law*, 24 (3) (1999), 421–88.

CHAPTER 2: CULTURE: DRUGS FOR ALL

15. T. De Quincey, *Confessions of an English Opium Eater*. First published 1821 (London: Penguin, 1971), 70–1.
16. De Quincey, *Confessions*, 71–2.
17. A. Hayter, *Opium and the Romantic Imagination* (London: Faber and Faber, 1968/71).
18. P. Wallis, 'Exotic drugs and English medicine: England's drug trade c.1550–c.1800', *Social History of Medicine*, 25 (1), (2012), 20–46.
19. Berridge, *Opium and the People*.
20. Quoted in Berridge, *Opium and the People*, 66.
21. 'Treatment of cholera at all the metropolitan hospitals', *Lancet* (1849) (2), 154.
22. Quoted in Berridge, *Opium and the People*, 68–9.
23. Quoted in Berridge, *Opium and the People*, 70–1.
24. Berridge, *Opium and the People*, 25–6.
25. Berridge, *Opium and the People*, 28.
26. 'Notes on Madras as a winter residence number III. Opium eating: districts of England in which it prevails, moral character of the English opium eater etc.', *Medical Times and Gazette*, 1873 (ii), 73.
27. The preceding sections are taken from Berridge, *Opium and the People*.
28. D. Courtwright, *Dark Paradise. Opiate Addiction in America before 1940* (Cambridge, MA: Harvard University Press, 1982).
29. David Courtwright, personal communication, 12 November 2012.
30. V. Berridge, 'Queen Victoria's cannabis use…', *Addiction Research and Theory*, 11 (4), (2003), 213–15.
31. Taken from P. Borsay, 'Bingeing Britain', *BBC History*, 6 (7), July 2005, 44–8.
32. R. Porter, 'The drinking man's disease: The "pre-history" of alcoholism in Georgian Britain', *British Journal of Addiction*, 80 (1985), 385–96.
33. Bamford 1849 quoted in P. Borsay, *A History of Leisure: The British Experience since 1500* (Basingstoke: Palgrave Macmillan, 2006).
34. Taken from evidence given to the House of Commons Health committee report on alcohol http://www.publications.parliament.uk/pa/cm200910/cmselect/cmhealth/151/15106.htm#n17 (last accessed 6 August 2013).
35. J. Macgregor, 'From dependence to binge: Drink in Nottingham from 1950 to the early twenty-first century', London University (LSHTM) PhD thesis, 2010, ch. 1. See also J. E. McGregor, *Drink and the City. Alcohol and Alcohol Problems in Urban UK since the 1950s*. (Nottingham: Nottingham University Press, 2012).
36. J. Goodman, *Tobacco in History*, 59.
37. Goodman, *Tobacco in History*, 85.

38. Quoted in M. Hilton, *Smoking in British Popular Culture, 1800–2000* (Manchester: Manchester University Press, 2000), 49.
39. M. Hilton, 'Smoking and sociability' in S. L. Gilman and Z. Xun, eds. *Smoke. A Global History of Smoking* (London: Reaktion Books, 2004), 126–33.

CHAPTER 3: SOCIAL MOVEMENTS: TEMPERANCE

40. Quoted in N. Longmate, *The Water Drinkers* (London: Hamish Hamilton, 1968), 43–4.
41. R. Porter, 'The drinking man's disease: The "pre-history" of alcoholism in Georgian Britain', *British Journal of Addiction*, 80 (1985), 385–96.
42. Quoted in Longmate, *The Water Drinkers*, 84.
43. B. Harrison, *Drink and the Victorians. The Temperance Question in England, 1815–1872* (Keele University Press reprint of Faber and Faber edn, 1971, 1994), 308.
44. Harrison, *Drink and the Victorians*, 123.
45. A. E. Dingle, *The Campaign for Prohibition in Victorian England* (London: Croom Helm, 1980), 205.
46. Quoted in Harrison, *Drink and the Victorians*, 115–16.
47. Harrison, *Drink and the Victorians*, 123.
48. Quoted in Longmate, *The Water Drinkers*, 123–4.
49. L. L. Shiman, *Crusade Against Drink in Victorian England* (Basingstoke: Macmillan, 1988), 124.
50. Quoted in Shiman, *Crusade Against Drink*, 152.
51. Quoted in Harrison, *Drink and the Victorians*, 28.
52. Dingle, *The Campaign for Prohibition*, 176–7 discusses its decline.
53. A. E. Dingle, 'The rise and fall of temperance economics', *Monash Papers in Economic History*, 3 (1977), 1–30.
54. Quoted in J. Greenaway, *Drink and British Politics since 1830. A Study in Policy Making* (Basingstoke: Palgrave Macmillan, 2003), 15.
55. Greenaway, *Drink and British Politics since 1830*, 88–9.
56. Longmate, *The Water Drinkers*, 236–7.
57. See also D. Gutzke, *Pubs and Progressives. Reinventing the Public House in Britain, 1896–1960* (DeKalb: Northern Illinois University Press, 2006).
58. I. R. Tyrrell, *Sobering Up. From Temperance to Prohibition in Ante bellum America, 1800–1860* (Westport Conn and London England: Greenwood Press, 1979), 13.
59. Tyrrell, *Sobering Up*, 11.
60. H. G. Levine, 'The alcohol problem in America: From temperance to alcoholism', *Addiction*, 79 (1984), 109–19.
61. Cited by H. G. Levine, 'Temperance cultures: Concern about alcohol problems in Nordic and English-speaking cultures' in M. Lader,

NOTES

G. Edwards, and C. Drummond, eds. *The Nature of Alcohol and Drug Related Problems* (Oxford: Oxford Medical Publications, 1992), 15–36.
62. Levine, 'The alcohol problem in America'.
63. Quoted in Berridge, *Opium and the People*, 187.
64. Quoted in Berridge, *Opium and the People*, 190.
65. R. B. Walker, 'Medical aspects of tobacco smoking and the anti-tobacco movement in Britain in the nineteenth century', *Medical History*, 24 (1980), 391–402.
66. M. Hilton and S. Nightingale, ' "A microbe of the devil's own make": Religion and science in the British anti-tobacco movement, 1853–1908' in S. Lock, L. Reynolds, and E. M.Tansey, eds. *Ashes to Ashes. The History of Smoking and Health* (Amsterdam: Rodopi, 1998), 41–77.

CHAPTER 4: THE PROFESSIONALS:
DOCTORS AND PHARMACISTS

67. Quoted from the Pharmacy in Practice oral history collection in S. Anderson and V. Berridge, 'Opium in 20th century Britain: pharmacists, regulation and the people', *Addiction*, 95(1), (2000), 23–36.
68. Oral history interviews and correspondence, quoted in V. Berridge, 'Opium and Oral History', *Oral History*, 72 (1979), 48–58.
69. Berridge, 118 quoting from Taylor's evidence to a House of Lords committee on the draft Pharmacy Bill.
70. Quoted Berridge, *Opium and the People*, 118–19.
71. Quoted Berridge, *Opium and the People*, 119.
72. A. Perry, *A Sunless Sea*. (London: Headline, 2012)
73. Quoted in Berridge, *Opium and the People*, 129.
74. Information from Bruno Bonnemain (France), Axel Helmstaedter (Germany) and Arjo Roersch van der Hoogte and Toine Pieters (Netherlands), the first two via Stuart Anderson.
75. Courtwright's assessment of the extent of addiction in *Dark Paradise* seems to imply that the prescription played an important role even within pharmacy. This was not the case in the UK until after the introduction of national health insurance in 1911.
76. Quoted in V. Berridge, 'The Society for the Study of Addiction, 1884–1988', special issue, *British Journal of Addiction*, 85 (8) (1990), 981–1088.
77. Quoted in V. Berridge, 'Punishment or treatment? Inebriety, drink and drugs, 1860–1914', *Lancet* , 364 (2004), 4–5.
78. The US historian David Courtwright states that the inebriety model also encompassed tobacco. This may have been the case in the US but was certainly not so in the UK.

79. H. Levine, 'The discovery of addiction. Changing conceptions of habitual drunkenness in America', *Journal of Studies on Alcohol*, 39 (1) (1978), 143–74.
80. Discussion in J. Nicholls, *The Politics of Alcohol*, 64–8.
81. Quoted in R. Porter, 'The drinking man's disease: The "pre-history" of alcoholism in Georgian Britain', *British Journal of Addiction*, 80 (1985), 385–96.
82. Taken from P. McCandless, ' "Curses of civilisation": Insanity and drunkenness in Victorian Britain', *British Journal of Addiction*, 79 (1984), 49–58.
83. W. B. Carpenter, *Temperance and Teetotalism. An Inquiry into the Effects of Alcoholic Drinks on the Human System in Health and Disease* (Glasgow: Scottish Temperance League, 1849), 19.
84. W. B. Carpenter, *On the Use and Abuse of Alcoholic Liquor in Health and Disease* (London: Charles Gilpin, 1850).
85. Discussed in Nicholls, *The Politics of Alcohol*, 170.
86. J. Woiak, ' "A medical Cromwell to depose King Alcohol": Cooperation and conflict between medical scientists and temperance reformers in Britain', *Histoire sociale/Social History*, 27 (1994), 337–65, reprinted in J. S. Blocker and C. K. Warsh, eds. *The Changing Face of Drink. Substance, Imagery, and Behaviour* (University of Ottawa Press, 1997), 237–70.
87. Analysis carried out for the FP7ALICE RAP workpackage on addiction through the ages.
88. Work carried out by Franca Beccaria and Enrico Petrilli for ALICE RAP workpackage.
89. W. White, *Slaying the Dragon. The History of Addiction Treatment and Recovery in America* (Bloomington Illinois: Chestnut Health Systems, 1998), 93.
90. Quoted in Berridge, *Opium and the People*, 163.
91. Quoted in S. Anderson, 'Community pharmacists and tobacco in Great Britain, from selling cigarettes to smoking cessation services', *Addiction*, 102 (2007), 704–12.
92. Harrison, *Drink and the Victorians*, 48.
93. M. Hilton, 'Constructing tobacco. Perspectives on consumer culture in Britain, 1850–1950', Lancaster PhD thesis, 1996.

CHAPTER 5: FEAR: DENS AND DEGENERATION

94. C. Dickens, *The Mystery of Edwin Drood*, first published 1870 (Harmondsworth: Penguin English library, 1974), 37.
95. G. Dore and B. Jerrold, *London, A Pilgrimage*, originally published 1872 (New York: Dover, 1970), 147–8.
96. O.Wilde, *The Picture of Dorian Gray*, first published 1891 (Harmondsworth: Penguin edn, 1966) 207–8.

97. A. Conan Doyle, "The man with the twisted lip", in *The Adventures of Sherlock Holmes* (London: George N. Newnes, 1892), originally published in *The Strand Magazine*, 1891.

98. G. Stedman Jones, *Outcast London. A Study in the Relationship between Classes in Victorian Society* (Oxford: Oxford University Press, 1971 and Peregrine Books, 1976).

99. Anon., 'London opium dens. Notes of a visit to the Chinaman's East End haunts. By a Social Explorer', *Good Words*, 26 (1885), 188–92, quoted in V. Berridge, 'East End opium dens and narcotic use in Britain', *London Journal*, 4 (1), (1978), 3–28.

100. *Good Words* quoted in Berridge, *London Journal*.

101. Quoted in Berridge, *London Journal*.

102. C.W. Wood, 'In the Night Watches', *Argosy* 65 (1897), 203 quoted in Berridge, *London Journal*.

103. Anon., 'Annual General Meeting', *Friend of China* 28 (1912), 222 quoted in Berridge, *London Journal*.

104. Interview by Virginia Berridge with Mr Cecil Limehouse quoted in Berridge, *London Journal*.

105. A. Lai, B. Little, and P. Little, 'Chinatown Annie: The East End opium trade, 1920–35: The story of a woman opium dealer', *Oral History* 14, 14 (1986), 18–26.

106. D. Ahmad, *The Opium Debate and Chinese Exclusion Laws in the Nineteenth-Century American West* (Reno and Las Vegas: University of Nevada Press, 2007), 27.

107. D. Musto, *The American Disease: Origins of Narcotic Control* (New Haven and London: Yale University Press, 1973), 7.

108. B. Milligan, *Pleasures and Pains. Opium and the Orient in Nineteenth-Century British Culture* (Charlottesville and London: University Press of Virginia, 1995), 93.

109. Quoted in Berridge (*London Journal*).

110. Quoted in W. Bynum, 'Alcoholism and degeneration in 19th-century European medicine and psychiatry', *British Journal of Addiction*, 79 (1984), 59–70, 62.

111. Sir V. Horsley and M. D. Sturge, *Alcohol and the Human Body* (London: Macmillan and Co, 1907), preface.

112. Quoted in J. Nicholls, *The Politics of Alcohol*, 174.

113. Quoted in V. Berridge 'The Society for the Study of Addiction, 1884–1988', special issue of *British Journal of Addiction*, 85 (8) (1990), 1002.

114. Quoted in Nicholls, *The Politics of Alcohol*, 173.

115. D.Gutzke, ' "The cry of the children": The Edwardian medical campaign against maternal drinking', *British Journal of Addiction*, 79 (1), (1984), 71–84.

116. Quoted in Gutzke, ' "The cry of the children"', 75.

117. Quoted in Gutzke, ' "The cry of the children"', 80.

118. Hilton, 'Constructing tobacco', 73–4.

CHAPTER 6: ECONOMICS AND TECHNOLOGY:
THE ROLE OF INDUSTRY

119. Courtwright, *Forces of Habit*, 9.
120. Burnett, *Liquid Pleasures*, 116.
121. P. Clark, *The English Alehouse. A Social History 1200–1830* (London: Longman, 1983), 293.
122. T. R. Gourvish and R. G. Wilson, *The British Brewing Industry, 1830–1980* (Cambridge: Cambridge University Press, 1994), 93.
123. Burnett, *Liquid Pleasures*, 117.
124. Burnett, *Liquid Pleasures*, 121–2.
125. K. Vernon, 'Pus, sewage, beer and milk: Microbiology in Britain, 1870–1940', *History of Science* 28 (1990), 289–325.
126. Gourvish and Wilson, *The British Brewing Industry, 1830–1980*, 100.
127. Burnett, *Liquid Pleasures*, 170.
128. Burnett, *Liquid Pleasures*, 120.
129. Greenaway, *Drink and British Politics since 1830*, 73–4.
130. D. Gutzke, *Protecting the Pub. Brewers and Publicans against Temperance* (Woodbridge: Royal Historical Society/Boydell and Brewer, 1989), 28–9.
131. G. B. Wilson, *Alcohol and the Nation. A Contribution to the Study of the Liquor Problem in the United Kingdom from 1800–1935* (London: Nicholson and Watson Ltd, 1940), 197.
132. Clark, *The English Alehouse*, 264.
133. Greenaway, *Drink and British Politics since 1830*, 58.
134. J. Rowntree and A. Sherwell, *The Temperance Problem and Social Reform* (London: Hodder and Stoughton, 1901).
135. Gutzke, *Protecting the Pub*, 51.
136. R. B. Weir, 'Obsessed with moderation: The drink trades and the drink question 1870–1930' *British Journal of Addiction*, 79(1),(1984), 93.
137. Greenaway, *Drink and British Politics since 1830*, 75, citing Wilson.
138. Rubinstein's calculations are cited in Gourvish and Wilson, *The British Brewing Industry, 1830–1980*, 217.
139. H. Cox, *The Global Cigarette. Origins and Evolution of British American Tobacco, 1880–1945* (Oxford: Oxford University Press, 2000), 3.
140. Quoted in B. Alford, *W.D. and H.O. Wills and the Development of the UK Tobacco Industry, 1786–1965* (London: Methuen and Co. Ltd, 1973) 146.
141. Brandt, *Cigarette Century*, 33–6.
142. Alford, *Development of the UK Tobacco Industry*, 314.
143. Hilton PhD thesis, 111–60, ch. 2.
144. Hilton, *Smoking in Popular Culture*, 89.
145. F. Dikotter, L. Laamann, and Z. Xun, *Narcotic Culture. A History of Drugs in China* (London: Hurst and Company, 2004), 202–3.

146. Quoted in Berridge, *Opium and the People*, 136.
147. Prescription book quoted in Berridge, *Opium and the People*, 138.
148. Quoted in Berridge, *Opium and the People*, 141.
149. Berridge, *Opium and the People*, 142.
150. Berridge, *Opium and the People*, 147.
151. Information from Stuart Anderson, citing H. N. Linstead, *Poisons Law* (London: The Pharmaceutical Press, 1936), 90.
152. Berridge, *Opium and the People*, 217.
153. J. F. Spillane, 'Making a modern drug: The manufacture, sale, and control of cocaine in the United States, 1880–1920' in P. Gootenberg, ed. *Cocaine. Global Histories* (London: Routledge, 1999), 21–45.
154. H. R. Friman, 'Germany and the transformation of cocaine, 1880–1920' in Gootenberg ed. *Cocaine*, 83–104.

CHAPTER 7: INTERNATIONALISM AND WAR

155. Letter from the Rt Revd Charles H. Brent, Protestant Episcopal bishop of the Philippine Islands cited in P. D. Lowes, *The Genesis of International Narcotics Control* (Geneva: Librarie Droz, 1966), 107–8.
156. N. Goodman, *International Health Organisations and their Work* (London: Churchill Livingstone, 1971).
157. N. Howard Jones, *The Scientific Background of the International Sanitary Conferences* (Geneva: WHO, 1975).
158. This section is based in general on V. Berridge, K. Loughlin, and R. Herring, 'Historical dimensions of global health governance' in K. Buse, W. Hein, and N. Drager, eds. *Making Sense of Global Health Governance. A Policy Perspective* (Basingstoke: Palgrave Macmillan, 2009), 28–46.
159. M. Harrison, annual lecture, Centre for History in Public Health, 2005.
160. There is discussion of this recent revisionist historiography in Dikotter, Laamann, and Xun, *Narcotic Culture*, especially 44–5.
161. J. Lovell, *The Opium War. Drugs, Dreams and the Making of China* (London: Picador, 2011), 359–67.
162. Report of the Royal Commission, quoted in Berridge, *Opium and the People*, 187.
163. Lowes, *The Genesis of International Narcotics Control*, 55.
164. William O. Walker III, '"A grave danger to the peace of the East": Opium and imperial rivalry in China, 1895–1920', in J. Mills and P. Barton, eds. *Drugs and Empires. Essays in Modern Imperialism and Intoxication, c1500–c1930* (Basingstoke: Palgrave Macmillan, 2007), 185–203, 188.
165. W. McAllister, *Drug Diplomacy in the Twentieth Century. An International History* (London: Routledge, 2000), 24–5.

166. Minute from Alston, 23 September 1909, in TNA, F.O.371/616/F241 The Foreign Office 371 series contains a very full discussion of the internal British government views on the US proposals, with comment from the India Office and Colonial Office.

167. Lowes, *The Genesis of International Narcotics Control*, 86.

168. Memorandum from Colonial Office to Foreign Office with additional material, 30 July 1910 TNA F.O.415/2 Further correspondence on opium.

169. India Office papers; Foreign Office papers FO371 and 415 and also Board of Trade papers BT11 quoted in Berridge, *Opium and the People*, 241–2.

170. Friman in Gootenberg, *Cocaine*, 83–104.

171. Report of the British delegates, cited by Berridge, *Opium and the People*, 242 and also FO refs.

172. Musto, *American Disease*, 121–50.

173. Berridge, *Opium and the People*, 246–9 and McAllister, *Drug Diplomacy*, 36.

174. Quoted in Berridge, *Opium and the People*, 252.

175. Committee on cocaine in dentistry quoted in Berridge, *Opium and the People*, 257.

176. Adams memorandum 1923, quoted in Berridge, *Opium and the People*, 273.

177. D. Downes, *Contrasts in Tolerance: Post War Penal Policy in the Netherlands and in England and Wales* (Oxford: Clarendon Press, 1988).

178. T. Brook and B.T. Wakabayashi, citing chapters by Brook and Motohiro, *Opium Regimes. China, Britain and Japan, 1839–1952* (Berkeley: University of California Press, 2000), 15–19.

179. A. A. Block, 'European drug traffic and traffickers between the wars: The policy of suppression and its consequences', *Journal of Social History*, 23 (2) (1989–90), 315–37.

180. J. Mills, 'Colonial Africa and the international politics of cannabis: Egypt, South Africa and the origins of global control' in Mills and Barton, eds. *Drugs and Empires*, 165–84.

181. Mills, 'Colonial Africa and the international politics of cannabis', 181.

182. McAllister, *Drug Diplomacy*, 77.

183. D. Bewley-Taylor, *The United States and International Drug Control, 1909–1997* (London: Pinter, 1999), 34–5.

184. A. W. McCoy, with C. B. Read and L. P. Adams II, *The Politics of Heroin in South East Asia* (New York: Harper and Rowe, 1972).

185. K. Bruun, L. Pan, and I. Rexed, *The Gentlemens' Club. International Control of Drugs and Alcohol* (Chicago and London: University of Chicago Press, 1975), 9, 12, and 165–73.

186. Hercod, speaking at International conference against Alcoholism, Geneva, 1925, quoted Bruun et al., 165.

187. This section based on J. Greenaway, *Drink and British Politics since 1830*, 129 onward.

188. Greenaway, *Drink and British Politics since 1830*, 106.

189. R. G. Smart, 'The effect of licensing restrictions during 1914–1918 on drunkenness and liver cirrhosis deaths in Britain', *British Journal of Addiction*, 69 (1974), 109–21.

190. I. Tyrrell, 'The US prohibition experiment: Myths, history and implications', *Addiction*, 92 (1997), 1405–9.

191. Jack S. Blocker, 'Did Prohibition really work? Alcohol prohibition as a public health innovation', *American Journal of Public Health*, 96 (2006), 233–43.

192. M. L. Schrad, *The Political Power of Bad Ideas. Networks, Institutions, and the Global Prohibition Wave* (New York: Oxford University Press, 2010).

CHAPTER 8: MASS CULTURE AND SUBCULTURE

193. Quoted in R. Elliot, *Women and Smoking since 1890* (London: Routledge, 2008), 45.

194. Quoted in P. Tinkler, *Smoke Signals. Women, Smoking and Visual Culture in Britain* (Oxford, Berg, 2006), 29.

195. *Daily Express*, 9 December 1918 quoted in M. Kohn, *Dope Girls. The Birth of the British Drug Underground* (London: Lawrence and Wishart, 1992), 105–6.

196. S. Rohmer, *Dope* (New York: McKinlay, Stone and Mackenzie, 1919), 117–18.

197. P. Tinkler, *Smoke Signals*, 42.

198. M. Hilton, *Smoking in Popular Culture*, 124.

199. Hilton, *Smoking in Popular Culture*, 125.

200. Information from Walter Holland, quoted in V. Berridge, *Marketing Health. Smoking and the Discourse of Public Health in Britain, 1945–2000* (Oxford: Oxford University Press, 2007), 47.

201. Elliot, *Women and Smoking since 1890*, 88.

202. Hilton, *Smoking in Popular Culture*, 130.

203. Quoted in Tinkler, *Smoke Signals*, 50.

204. Quoted in Elliot, *Women and Smoking since 1890*, 81.

205. Quoted in Elliot, *Women and Smoking since 1890*, 108.

206. L. Jeger, 'The social implications' in C. Fletcher, H. Cole, L. Jeger, and C. Wood, *Common Sense about Smoking* (Harmondsworth: Penguin special, 1963), 93–4.

207. A. Brandt, 'Recruiting women smokers: The engineering of consent', *Journal of the American Womens' Association*, 51 (1996), 63–6.

208. Brandt, *Cigarette Century*, 78.

209. A. Bingham, *Gender, Modernity and the Popular Press in Inter War Britain* (Oxford, Clarendon Press 2004).
210. Tinkler, *Smoke Signals*, 7, 11, 57, 59.
211. Quoted in V. Berridge, 'The origins of the English drug "scene"', *Medical History*, 32 (1988), 51–64.
212. Symons, Poems, quoted in Berridge, 'Drug scene', 55.
213. Weir Mitchell quoted in Berridge, 57.
214. M. Pugh, *'We Danced all Night'. A Social History of Britain between the Wars* (London: The Bodley Head, 2008), 159.
215. *Daily Express*, 11 March 1922.
216. *Daily Express*, 4 May 1922 and TNA Home Office papers HO45/11599.
217. *Times*, 8 April 1922, quoted in T. Parssinen, *Secret Passions, Secret Remedies. Narcotic Drugs in British Society, 1800–1926* (Manchester: Manchester University Press, 1983), 173.
218. Parssinen, *Secret Passions, Secret Remedies*, 178.
219. Pugh, *'We Danced all Night'*, 217.
220. Interview with Mr Cecil, quoted in Berridge, 'Opium den', 9.
221. TNA Home Office papers HO45/432886/17a Henderson case 21 November 1922.
222. Ziegler, quoted in Berridge, 'Drug scene', 61.
223. Quoted in M. Pugh, *'We Danced all Night'*, 45.
224. Crowley, 1922, cited in Berridge, 'Drug scene', 63.
225. Wishart quoted in P. Hoare DNB entry for Brenda Dean Paul.
226. D, Courtwright, *Dark Paradise. Opiate Addiction in America before 1940* (London: Harvard University Press, 1982), 113.
227. Courtwright, *Dark Paradise*, 124.
228. Mel quoted in D. Courtwright, H. Joseph, and D. Des Jarlais, *Addicts who Survived. An Oral History of Narcotic Use in America, 1923–1965* (Knoxville: University of Tennessee Press, 1989), 88.

CHAPTER 9: THE NEW PUBLIC HEALTH

229. House of Commons Health Committee. *First Report on Alcohol* session 2009–10.
230. J. Collins paper given at LSHTM autumn 2012.
231. Jerry Morris, 'Coronary thrombosis: A modern epidemic', *The Listener*, 8 December 1955, 995–6, quoted in Berridge, *Marketing Health*, 61.
232. R. Doll, 'The first reports on smoking and lung cancer' in S. Lock, L. Reynolds, and E. M. Tansey, *Ashes to Ashes: The History of Smoking and Health* (Amsterdam: Rodopi, 1998), 130–40.

233. 'Conversation with Sir Richard Doll', *British Journal of Addiction*, 86 (4) (1991), 365–77.
234. TNA Ministry of Health papers MH55/1011 Letter from Ian Macleod to John Boyd Carpenter, 29 January 1954.
235. Fletcher in Lock et al., 203.
236. Cited in Berridge, *Marketing Health*, 196.
237. TNA Ministry of Health papers MH 55/2204 Minute from Enid Russell Smith 5 February 1962. Quoted in Berridge, *Marketing Health*, 167.
238. Wellcome Library London ASH archive SA/ASH William Norman collection R.12 Box 77. Interview with Mike Daube, quoted in Berridge, *Marketing Health*, 173.
239. Royal College of Physicians, *Smoking or Health*. The Third Report from the Royal College of Physicians of London (London: Pitman Medical, 1977), 27, quoted in Berridge, 176.
240. Interview with Mike Daube by Virginia Berridge 11 March 1999, quoted Berridge, *Marketing Health*, 174.
241. Cited in Berridge, *Marketing Health*, 121.
242. TNA Ministry of Health MH55/2221 papers quoted in NSNS publicity material sent to the Ministry. Quoted in Berridge, *Marketing Health*, 217.
243. Independent Scientific Committee on Smoking and Health (ISCSH) *Fourth Report of the Independent Scientific Committee on Smoking and Health* (London: HMSO, 1988) quoted in Berridge, 222.
244. M. Hilton, 'Smoking and Sociability' in S. Gilman and Z. Xun, eds. *Smoke. A Global History of* Smoking (London: Reaktion Books, 2004), 126–33.
245. Quoted in Berridge, *Marketing Health*, 229.
246. B. Jacobson, *Beating the Ladykillers* (London: Gollancz, 1988), 138, quoted in Berridge, *Marketing Health*, 231–2.
247. Interview with Alan Marsh by Virginia Berridge, 3 November 1997 quoted in Berridge, *Marketing Health*, 256.
248. Graham's work is cited in Berridge, *Marketing Health*, 232–3.
249. Wellcome Library, ASH archive Box 79 R.30 Rights of the non smoker, 1975–7, quoted in Berridge, *Marketing Health*, 228.
250. P. Froggatt, 'Determinants of Policy on Smoking and Health', *International Journal of Epidemiology*, 18 (1), (1989), 1–9 quoted in Berridge, *Marketing Health*, 215.
251. Nathanson, 'Social movements', 471.
252. R. Elliot, 'Smoking for taxation: The triumph of fiscal policy over health in postwar West Germany, 1945–55', *Economic History Review* online 29 February 2012.

253. Wellcome Library. ASH archive William Norman papers. R.18 Box 77. Godber file. Godber's speech to third world conference on smoking and health., quoted in Berridge, *Marketing Health*, 235.

CHAPTER 10: CONVERGENCE OR DIVERGENCE?
PUBLIC HEALTH AND NEUROSCIENCE

254. L. N. Robins, 'Vietnam veterans' rapid recovery from heroin addiction: A fluke or normal expectation?', *Addiction*, 88 (8), (1993), 1037–67.
255. Interview with Dr Jerry Jaffe http://www.pbs.org/wgbh/pages/frontline/ shows/drugs/interviews/jaffe.html (last accessed 6 August 2013).
256. K. Bruun, G. Edwards, M. Lumio et al., *Alcohol Control Policies in Public Health Perspective* (Helsinki: Finnish Foundation for Alcohol Studies, 1975).
257. A. Mold, *Heroin. The Treatment of Addiction in Twentieth-Century Britain* (De Kalb: Northern Illinois University Press, 2008).
258. R. Hartnoll, R. Lewis, M. Mitcheson, et al., 'Estimating the prevalence of opioid dependence', *Lancet*, 26 January 1985, 203–5.
259. McClelland report 1986. *HIV Infection in Scotland: Report of the Scottish Committee on HIV Infection and Intravenous Drug Misuse* (Edinburgh: Scottish Home and Health Department, 1986).
260. R. Room, 'The World Health Organisation and alcohol control', *British Journal of Addiction*, 79 (1) (1984), 85–92.
261. Royal College of Physicians, *Smoking and Health Now* (London: Pitman, 1971).
262. G. Edwards, M. A. H. Russell, D. Hawks, and M. Macafferty, eds. *Alcohol Dependence and Smoking Behaviour* (Farnborough: Saxon House and Lexington Books, 1976), 205–6 quoted Berridge, *Marketing Health*, 261.
263. Interview with smoking psychologist by Virginia Berridge, 26 June 1996, quoted in Berridge, *Marketing Health*, 263.
264. Quoted in G. Stimson, 'Research on British drug policy' in V. Berridge, ed. *Drugs Research and Policy in Britain* (Aldershot: Avebury, 1990), 266.
265. Quoted in Berridge, *Marketing Health*, 272.
266. D. Healy, *The Anti-Depressant Era* (Cambridge, MA and London: Harvard University Press, 1997).
267. J. Hughes, 'The nature of addiction: The pharmacological approach' in V. Berridge, ed. *Drugs Research and Policy in Britain*, 237–59.
268. Interview with psychopharmacologist by Virginia Berridge, 1995.
269. A. Goldstein, *Addiction. From Biology to Drug Policy* (Oxford: Oxford University Press, 2001), 2nd edn; the 1st edn (1993) has a section on 'The drugs and the addicts' which brings all these substances together.

270. A. K. Armitage and G. H. Hall, 'Further evidence relating to the mode of action of nicotine in the central nervous system', *Nature*, 214 (1967), 977.
271. A. K. Armitage and C. F. Morrison, 'Pharmacological basis for the tobacco smoking habit', *Nature*, 217 (1968), 331.
272. Royal College of Physicians (RCP) archive, tobacco committee minutes May 1967.
273. RCP archive May 1967.
274. Sir P. Froggatt and N. Wald, 'The role of nicotine in the tar reduction programme' in N. Wald and P. Froggatt, eds. *Nicotine Smoking and the Low Tar Programme* (Oxford: Oxford University Press, 1989), 229–35, quoted in Berridge, *Marketing Health*, 275.
275. C. Snowdon, *Velvet Glove, Iron Fist* (UK: Little Dice, 2009), 190 onward.
276. Quoted in A. Mold and V. Berridge, *Voluntary Action and Illegal Drugs. Health and Society in Britain since the 1960s* (Basingstoke: Palgrave Macmillan, 2010), 145.
277. V. Berridge, 'AIDS and British drug policy: Continuity or change?' in V. Berridge and P. Strong, eds. *AIDS and Contemporary History* (Cambridge: Cambridge University Press, 1993), 135–56.
278. R. Proctor, *Golden Holocaust. Origins of the Cigarette Catastrophe and the Case for Abolition* (Berkeley: University of California Press, 2011).
279. Russell, *Lancet*, 1991, quoted in Berridge, *Marketing Health*, 271–2.
280. J. Le Houezec, A. McNeill and J. Britton, 'Tobacco, nicotine and harm reduction', *Drug and Alcohol Review* (March, 2011), 30, 119–23.
281. C. E. Gartner, A. Carter, and B. Partridge, 'What are the public policy implications of a neuro biological view of addiction?' *Addiction*, 107 (7) (2012), 1199–1200.
282. Email from Monica Guarinoni senior policy advisor Milieu Ltd to Dr Sandra Mounier Jack, LSHTM, 7 March 2013.
283. J. Greene, *Prescribing by Numbers. Drugs and the Definition of Disease* (Baltimore; John Hopkins University Press, 2007).
284. Paper by Jim Orford about the early brief intervention work, Edwards memorial conference, Institute of Psychiatry, 24 January 2013.
285. Report of the Committee on the Safety of Medicines working party on Nicotine Replacement Therapy 2005.
286. Becker and Murphy, 1988, quoted in Berridge, *Marketing Health*, 265.
287. T. Hickman, 'Target America: Visual culture, neuroimaging and the "hijacked brain" theory of addiction', paper at LSHTM 2011.
288. Sir D. King, 'Introduction' in D. Nutt, T. Robbins, G.V. Stimson, M. Ince, and A. Jackson, *Drugs and the Future. Brain Science, Addiction and Society* (London: Elsevier, 2007), xi.

289. D. Courtwright, 'Mr ATOD's wild ride: What do alcohol, tobacco, and other drugs have in common?', *Social History of Alcohol and Drugs*, 20 (2005), 105–40.

CHAPTER 11: HEDONISM OR CONTROL?

290. Berridge, cannabis article *Addiction Research and Theory*.
291. This section is based on L. Iversen, 'Introduction' and S. Taylor comments in S. M. Crowther, L. A. Reynolds, and E. M. Tansey, eds. *The Medicalisation of Cannabis* (London: Wellcome Trust, 2010) and on the University of London PhD thesis by S.Taylor on the same topic, 2010.
292. R. Room, B. Fischer, W.Hall, S. Lenton, and P. Reuter, *Cannabis Policy. Moving Beyond Stalemate* (Oxford: Beckley Foundation/Oxford University Press, 2010).
293. Taken from E. Dyck, *Psychedelic Psychiatry. LSD from Clinic to Campus* (Baltimore: Johns Hopkins University Press, 2008).
294. Beckley Foundation email of 8 February 2012 drawing on *Guardian* science report 6 February 2012.
295. National Treatment Agency, *Injectable Heroin (and Injectable Methadone): Potential Roles in Drug Treatment* (London: NTA, 2003).
296. EMCDDA, *New Heroin Assisted Treatment. Recent Evidence and Current Practices of Supervised Injectable Heroin Treatment in Europe and Beyond* (Lisbon: EMCDDA, 2012).
297. Presentation by Les King at EMCDDA conference Lisbon, 2009.
298. D. Nutt, T. Robbins, and G. Stimson, 'Drugs futures 2025' in Nutt, Robbins, Stimson et al., *Foresight*, 2007.
299. P. Butler, ' "Hidden" drug users who won't be found burgling your home to fund their habit', *Guardian*, 15 March 2012.
300. J. Greene, *Prescribing by Numbers*, 2007.
301. C. Snowden, *Velvet Glove, Iron Fist*, 211, 271–2.
302. M. Elam and A, Gunnarsson, 'The advanced liberal logic of nicotine replacement and the Swedish invention of smoking as addiction' in B. Larsson, M. Letell, and H. Thorn, eds. *Transformations of the Swedish Welfare State: From Social Engineering to Governance?* (London: Palgrave Macmillan, 2012).
303. Author's notes from NDT conference, 2006.
304. C. Brewer, 'Ten years on', *Druglink*, 17 March/April 2012, 16–17.
305. A. Gilmore and M. McKee, 'Tobacco control policy in the European Union' in E. Feldman and R.Bayer, eds. *Unfiltered. Conflicts over Tobacco Policy and Public Health* (Cambridge: Harvard University Press, 2004), 219–54.

306. Joy Townsend, interview with David Reubi, LSHTM, 2010.
307. Analysed in Mold and Berridge *Voluntary Action and Illegal Drugs. Health and Society in Britain since the 1960s* (Basingstoke: Palgrave Macmillan, 2010).
308. Nordic researchers quoted by Mold and Berridge, p. 164.
309. J. Collins presentation, 2012.
310. R. Room and P. Reuter, 'How well do international drug conventions protect public health?', *Lancet*, 379, 7 January 2012, 84–91.
311. V. Berridge, 'Introduction' in L. A. Reynolds and E. M. Tansey, eds. *WHO Framework Convention on Tobacco Control* (London: QMUL, 2012).
312. Gilmore and McKee in *Unfiltered*.
313. J. Macgregor book and PhD thesis.
314. V. Berridge, R. Herring, and B. Thom, *The Normalisation of Binge Drinking? A Historical and Cross Cultural Investigation with Implications for Action* (London: Alcohol Education and Research Council, 2007).
315. Berridge, Herring, and Thom and V. Berridge, *Temperance: Its History and Impact on Current and Future Alcohol Policy* (York: JRF, 2005).
316. K. Lowe and E. J. Lee, 'Advocating alcohol abstinence to pregnant women: Some observations about British policy', *Health, Risk and Society*, 12(4) (2010), 301–11.
317. KBS email correspondence.
318. Comment at ALRUK meeting, 2012.
319. J. Rutter, E. Marshall, and S. Sims, *The 'S' Factor. Lessons from IFG's Policy Success Reunions* (London: Institute for Government 2012).
320. Owen interview cited in Berridge, *Marketing Health*, 149–50.
321. D. Carpenter, *Reputation and Power. Organisational Image and Pharmaceutical Regulation at the FDA* (Princeton and Oxford: Princeton University Press, 2010).
322. R. J. MacCoun and P. Reuter, *Drug War Heresies. Learning from other Vices, Times and Places* (Cambridge: Cambridge University Press, 2001).
323. D. Bewley-Taylor *International Drug Control. Consensus Fractured.* (Cambridge: Cambridge University Press, 2012).
324. Ministry of Justice, *Sentencing Statistics: England and Wales 2009* (London: Ministry of Justice, 2010).
325. ACMD 2005 report on khat quoted in S. Beckerleg, *Ethnic Identity and Development. Khat and Social Change in Africa* (Basingstoke: Palgrave Macmillan, 2010).
326. D. Anderson, S. Beckerleg, D. Hailu, and A. Klein, *The Khat Controversy. Stimulating the Debate on Drugs* (Oxford: Berg, 2007), 10.

CHAPTER 12: AFTERWORD: HISTORY AND THE FUTURE

327. D. Nutt, *Drugs without the Hot Air. Minimising the Harms of Legal and Illegal Drugs* (Cambridge, UIT, 2012).
328. S. Pryce, *Fixing Drugs. The Politics of Drug Prohibition* (Basingstoke: Palgrave Macmillan, 2012).
329. P. Bean, *Legalising Drugs. Debates and Dilemmas* (Bristol: Policy Press, 2010).
330. N. McKeganey, *Controversies in Drug Policy and Practice* (Basingstoke: Palgrave Macmillan, 2011).
331. Jayne C. Luck and Wayne D. Hall, 'Under what conditions is it ethical to encourage drug-using women to use long acting forms of contraception?', *Addiction*, online 11 February 2012.
332. R. Room, B. Fischer, W. Hall, S. Lenton, and P. Reuter, *Cannabis Policy. Moving Beyond Stalemate* (Oxford: Beckley Foundation/Oxford University Press, 2010).

FURTHER READING

Listed below are some of the books and articles I have found most helpful in writing the book. The in-depth historiographical framework on which I have drawn for parts of it is to be found in my *Opium and the People. Opiate Use and Drug Control Policy in Nineteenth and Early Twentieth-Century England* (London: Free Association Books, 1999), expanded edn; *AIDS in the UK. The Making of Policy, 1981–1994* (Oxford: Oxford University Press, 1996); *Marketing Health: Smoking and the Discourse of Public Health in Britain, 1945–2000* (Oxford: Oxford University Press, 2007), and other articles and reports on the substances, including alcohol.

CHAPTER 1: INTRODUCTION: PAST AND PRESENT

Berridge, V. *Opium and the People. Opiate Use and Drug Control Policy in Nineteenth and Early Twentieth-Century England* (London: Free Association Books, 1999), expanded edn.

Burnett, J. *Liquid Pleasures. A Social History of Drinks in Modern Britain* (London: Routledge, 1999).

Courtwright, D. *Forces of Habit. Drugs and the Making of the Modern World* (Cambridge, MA: Harvard University Press, 2001).

Goodman, J. *Tobacco in History. The Cultures of Dependence* (London: Routledge, 1993).

Goodman, J., P. E. Lovejoy, and A. Sherratt, eds. *Consuming Habits. Global and Historical Perspectives on How Cultures Define Drugs* (Abingdon: Routledge, 2007), 2nd edn.

Nicholls, J. *The Politics of Alcohol. A History of the Drink Question in England* (Manchester: Manchester University Press, 2009).

Nutt, D., L. A. King, W. Saulsbury, and C. Blakemore, 'Development of a rational scale to assess the harm of drugs of potential misuse', *Lancet*, 369 (2007), 1047–53.

CHAPTER 2: CULTURE: DRUGS FOR ALL

Borsay, P. *A History of Leisure: The British Experience since 1500* (Basingstoke: Palgrave Macmillan, 2006).

Courtwright, D. *Dark Paradise. Opiate Addiction in America before 1940* (Cambridge, MA: Harvard University Press, 1982).

De Quincey T. *Confessions of an English Opium Eater.* First published 1821 (London: Penguin, 1971).

Gilman S. L., and Z. Xun, *Smoke. A Global History of Smoking* (London: Reaktion Books, 2004).

Hayter, A. *Opium and the Romantic Imagination* (London: Faber and Faber, 1968/71).

Hilton, M. *Smoking in British Popular Culture, 1800–2000* (Manchester: Manchester University Press, 2000).

Evidence given to the House of Commons Health committee report on alcohol http://www.publications.parliament.uk/pa/cm200910/cmselect/cmhealth/151/15106.htm#n17.

CHAPTER 3: SOCIAL MOVEMENTS: TEMPERANCE

Dingle, A. E. *The Campaign for Prohibition in Victorian England* (London: Croom Helm, 1980).

Greenaway, J. *Drink and British Politics since 1830. A Study in Policy Making* (Basingstoke: Palgrave Macmillan, 2003).

Gutzke, D. *Pubs and Progressives. Reinventing the Public House in Britain, 1896–1960* (DeKalb: Northern Illinois University Press, 2006).

Harrison, B. *Drink and the Victorians. The Temperance Question in England, 1815–1872* (Keele: Keele University Press reprint of Faber and Faber edn, 1971, 1994).

Hilton, M. and S. Nightingale, '"A microbe of the devil's own make": Religion and science in the British anti tobacco movement, 1853–1908' in S. Lock, L. Reynolds, and E. M. Tansey, eds. *Ashes to Ashes. The History of Smoking and Health* (Amsterdam: Rodopi, 1998), 41–77.

Levine, H. G. 'The alcohol problem in America: From temperance to alcoholism', *Addiction*, 79 (1984), 109–19.

Longmate, N. *The Water Drinkers* (London: Hamish Hamilton, 1968).

Tyrrell, I. R. *Sobering Up. From Temperance to Prohibition in Ante bellum America, 1800–1860* (Westport, CT and London England: Greenwood Press, 1979).

CHAPTER 4: THE PROFESSIONALS:
DOCTORS AND PHARMACISTS

Anderson, S. 'Community pharmacists and tobacco in Great Britain, from selling cigarettes to smoking cessation services', *Addiction*, 102 (2007), 704–12.

Berridge, V. 'Punishment or treatment? Inebriety, drink and drugs, 1860–1914', *Lancet*, 364 (2004), 4–5.

Levine, H. 'The discovery of addiction. Changing conceptions of habitual drunkenness in America', *Journal of Studies on Alcohol*, 39 (1) (1978), 143–74.

Porter, R. 'The drinking man's disease: the "pre-history" of alcoholism in Georgian Britain', *British Journal of Addiction*, 80 (1985), 385–96.

White, W. *Slaying the Dragon. The History of Addiction Treatment and Recovery in America* (Bloomington Illinois: Chestnut Health Systems, 1998).

Woiak, J. '"A medical Cromwell to depose King Alcohol": Cooperation and conflict between medical scientists and temperance reformers in Britain', *Histoire sociale/Social history*, 27 (1994), 337–65, reprinted in J. S Blocker and C. K. Warsh, eds. *The Changing Face of Drink: Substance, Imagery, and Behaviour* (University of Ottawa Press, 1997), 237–70.

CHAPTER 5: FEAR: DENS AND DEGENERATION

Ahmad, D. *The Opium Debate and Chinese Exclusion Laws in the Nineteenth-Century American West* (Reno and Las Vegas: University of Nevada Press, 2007).

Berridge, V. 'East End opium dens and narcotic use in Britain', *London Journal*, 4 (1) (1978), 3–28.

Berridge, V. 'The Society for the Study of Addiction, 1884–1988', special issue of *British Journal of Addiction*, 85 (8) (1990), 983–1087.

Bynum, W. 'Alcoholism and degeneration in 19th-century European medicine and psychiatry', *British Journal of Addiction*, 79 (1984), 59–70.

Dickens, C. *The Mystery of Edwin Drood*, first published 1870 (Harmondsworth: Penguin English Library, 1974).

Gutzke, D. '"The cry of the children": The Edwardian medical campaign against maternal drinking', *British Journal of Addiction*, 79 (1) (1984), 71–84.

Lai, A., B. Little and P. Little, 'Chinatown Annie: The East End opium trade, 1920–35: The story of a women opium dealer', *Oral History*, 14 (1986), 18–26.

Milligan, B. *Pleasures and Pains. Opium and the Orient in Nineteenth-Century British Culture* (Charlottesville and London: University Press of Virginia, 1995).

Musto, D. *The American Disease: Origins of Narcotic Control* (New Haven and London: Yale University Press, 1973).

Wilde, O. *The Picture of Dorian Gray*, first published 1891 (Harmondsworth: Penguin edn, 1966).

CHAPTER 6: ECONOMICS AND TECHNOLOGY: THE ROLE OF INDUSTRY

Alford, B. *W.D. and H. O. Wills and the Development of the UK Tobacco Industry, 1786–1965* (London: Methuen and Co. Ltd, 1973).

Brandt, A. *The Cigarette Century: The Rise, Fall and Deadly Persistence of the Product that Defined America* (New York: Basic Books, 2007).

Clark, P. *The English Alehouse. A Social History 1200–1830* (London: Longman, 1983).

Cox, H. *The Global Cigarette. Origins and Evolution of British American Tobacco, 1880–1945* (Oxford: Oxford University Press, 2000).

Dikotter, F., L. Laamann, and Z. Xun, *Narcotic Culture. A History of Drugs in China* (London: Hurst and Company, 2004).

Gootenberg, P., ed. *Cocaine. Global Histories* (London: Routledge, 1999).

Gourvish T. R. and R. G. Wilson, *The British Brewing Industry, 1830–1980* (Cambridge: Cambridge University Press, 1994).

Gutzke, D. *Protecting the Pub. Brewers and Publicans against Temperance* (Woodbridge: Royal Historical Society/Boydell and Brewer, 1989).

Wilson, G. B. *Alcohol and the Nation. A Contribution to the Study of the Liquor Problem in the United Kingdom from 1800–1935* (London: Nicholson and Watson Ltd, 1940).

CHAPTER 7: INTERNATIONALISM AND WAR

Berridge, V., K. Loughlin, and R. Herring, 'Historical dimensions of global health governance' in K. Buse, W. Hein, and N. Drager, eds. *Making Sense of Global Health Governance. A Policy Perspective* (Basingstoke: Palgrave Macmillan, 2009), 28–46.

Bewley-Taylor, D. *The United States and International Drug Control, 1909–1997* (London: Pinter, 1999).

Block, A. A. 'European drug traffic and traffickers between the wars: The policy of suppression and its consequences', *Journal of Social History*, 23 (2) (1989–90), 315–37.

Blocker, Jack S. 'Did Prohibition really work? Alcohol prohibition as a public health innovation', *American Journal of Public Health*, 96 (2006), 233–43.

Brook T. and B. T. Wakabayashi, citing chapters by Brook and Motohiro, *Opium Regimes. China, Britain and Japan, 1839–1952* (Berkeley: University of California Press, 2000).

Bruun, K., L. Pan and I. Rexed, *The Gentlemens' Club. International Control of Drugs and Alcohol* (Chicago and London: University of Chicago Press, 1975).

Lovell, J. *The Opium War. Drugs, Dreams and the Making of China* (London: Picador, 2011).

Lowes, P. D. *The Genesis of International Narcotics Control* (Geneva: Librarie Droz, 1966).

McAllister, W. *Drug Diplomacy in the Twentieth Century. An International History* (London: Routledge, 2000).

McCoy, A. W. with C. B. Read and L. P. Adams II, *The Politics of Heroin in South East Asia* (New York: Harper and Rowe, 1972).

Mills, J. 'Colonial Africa and the international politics of Cannabis: Egypt, South Africa and the origins of global control' in Mills and Barton, eds. *Drugs and Empires* (2007), 165–84.

Schrad, M. L. *The Political Power of Bad Ideas. Networks, Institutions, and the Global Prohibition Wave* (New York: Oxford University Press, 2010).

Smart, R. G. 'The effect of licensing restrictions during 1914–1918 on drunkenness and liver cirrhosis deaths in Britain', *British Journal of Addiction*, 69 (1974), 109–21.

Tyrrell, I. 'The US prohibition experiment: Myths, history and implications', *Addiction*, 92 (1997), 1405–9.

Walker III, W. O. '"A grave danger to the peace of the east": Opium and imperial rivalry in China, 1895–1920' in Mills and Barton, eds. *Drugs and Empires* (2007), 188 in 185–203.

CHAPTER 8: MASS CULTURE AND SUB CULTURE

Berridge, V. *Marketing Health. Smoking and the Discourse of Public Health in Britain, 1945–2000* (Oxford: Oxford University Press, 2007).

Courtwright, D., H. Joseph and D. Des Jarlais, *Addicts who Survived. An Oral History of Narcotic Use in America, 1923–1965* (Knoxville: University of Tennessee Press, 1989).

Elliot, R. *Women and Smoking since 1890* (London: Routledge, 2008).

Kohn, M. *Dope Girls. The Birth of the British Drug Underground* (London: Lawrence and Wishart, 1992).

Parssinen, T. *Secret Passions, Secret Remedies. Narcotic Drugs in British Society, 1800–1926* (Manchester: Manchester University Press, 1983).

Pugh, M. *'We Danced all Night'. A Social History of Britain Between the Wars* (London: The Bodley Head, 2008).

Tinkler, P. *Smoke Signals. Women, Smoking and Visual Culture in Britain* (Oxford: Berg, 2006).

CHAPTER 9: THE NEW PUBLIC HEALTH

Berridge, V. *Marketing Health. Smoking and the Discourse of Public Health in Britain, 1945–2000* (Oxford: Oxford University Press, 2007).

Elliot, R. 'Smoking for taxation: The triumph of fiscal policy over health in postwar West Germany, 1945–51', *Economic History Review*, 65 (4) (2012), 145–74.

Lock, S., L. Reynolds, and E. M. Tansey, *Ashes to Ashes: The History of Smoking and Health* (Amsterdam: Rodopi, 1998).

CHAPTER 10: CONVERGENCE OR DIVERGENCE?
PUBLIC HEALTH AND NEUROSCIENCE

Berridge, V. ed. *Drugs Research and Policy in Britain* (Aldershot: Avebury, 1990)

Berridge, V. 'AIDS and British Drug Policy: continuity or change?' in V. Berridge and P. Strong, eds. *AIDS and Contemporary History* (Cambridge: Cambridge University Press, 1993), 135–56.

Bruun, K., G. Edwards, M. Lumio et al., *Alcohol Control Policies in Public Health Perspective* (Helsinki: Finnish Foundation for Alcohol Studies, 1975).

Courtwright, D. 'Mr ATOD's wild ride: What do alcohol, tobacco, and other drugs have in common?', *Social History of Alcohol and Drugs*, 20 (2005), 105–40.

Greene, J. *Prescribing by Numbers. Drugs and the Definition of Disease* (Baltimore: John Hopkins University Press, 2007).

Healy, D. *The Anti-Depressant Era* (Cambridge, MA and London: Harvard University Press, 1997).

Mold, A. *Heroin. The Treatment of Addiction in Twentieth-Century Britain* (De Kalb: Northern Illinois University Press, 2008).

Mold, A. and V. Berridge, *Voluntary Action and Illegal Drugs. Health and Society in Britain since the 1960s* (Basingstoke: Palgrave Macmillan, 2010).

Nutt, D., T. Robbins, G.V Stimson, M. Ince, and A. Jackson, *Drugs and the Future. Brain Science, Addiction and Society* (London: Elsevier, 2007).

Proctor, R. *Golden Holocaust: Origins of the Cigarette Catastrophe and the Case for Abolition* (Berkeley: University of California Press, 2011).

Robins, L. N. 'Vietnam veterans' rapid recovery from heroin addiction: A fluke or normal expectation?', *Addiction*, 88 (8) (1993), 1037–67.

Room, R. 'The World Health Organisation and alcohol control', *British Journal of Addiction*, 79 (1) (1984), 85–92.

Snowdon, C. *Velvet Glove, Iron Fist* (UK: Little Dice, 2009).

CHAPTER 11: HEDONISM OR CONTROL?

Anderson, D., S. Beckerleg, D. Hailu, and A. Klein, *The Khat Controversy. Stimulating the Debate on Drugs* (Oxford: Berg, 2007).

Beckerleg, S. *Ethnic Identity and Development. Khat and Social Change in Africa* (Basingstoke: Palgrave Macmillan, 2010).

Berridge, V. *Temperance: Its History and Impact on Current and Future Alcohol Policy* (York: JRF, 2005).

Berridge, V., R. Herring, and B. Thom, *The Normalisation of Binge Drinking? A Historical and Cross Cultural Investigation with Implications for Action* (London: Alcohol Education and Research Council, 2007).

Berridge, V. 'Introduction' in L. A. Reynolds and E. M. Tansey, eds. *WHO Framework Convention on Tobacco Control* (London: QMUL, 2012).

Bewley-Taylor, D. *International Drug Control. Consensus Fractured* (Cambridge: Cambridge University Press, 2012).

Carpenter, D. *Reputation and Power. Organisational Image and Pharmaceutical Regulation at the FDA* (Princeton and Oxford: Princeton University Press, 2010).

Crowther, S. M., L. A. Reynolds, and E. M. Tansey, eds. *The Medicalisation of Cannabis* (London: Wellcome Trust, 2010).

Dyck, E. *Psychedelic Psychiatry. LSD from Clinic to Campus* (Baltimore: Johns Hopkins University Press, 2008).

EMCDDA, *New Heroin Assisted Treatment. Recent Evidence and Current Practices of Supervised Injectable Heroin Treatment in Europe and Beyond* (Lisbon: EMCDDA, 2012)

Gilmore, A. and M. McKee, 'Tobacco control policy in the European Union' in E. Feldman and R. Bayer, eds. *Unfiltered. Conflicts over Tobacco Policy and Public Health* (Cambridge: Harvard University Press, 2004), 219–54.

MacCoun, R. J. and P. Reuter, *Drug War Heresies. Learning from other Vices, Times and Places* (Cambridge: Cambridge University Press, 2001).

Room, R. and P. Reuter, 'How well do international drug conventions protect public health?', *Lancet*, 379, 7 January 2012, 84–91.

Rutter, J., E. Marshall, and S. Sims, *The 'S' Factor. Lessons from IFG's Policy Success Reunions* (London: Institute for Government, 2012).

CHAPTER 12: AFTERWORD: HISTORY AND THE FUTURE

Bean, P. *Legalising Drugs. Debates and Dilemmas* (Bristol: Policy Press, 2010).

McKeganey, N. *Controversies in Drug Policy and Practice* (Basingstoke: Palgrave Macmillan, 2011).

Nutt, D. *Drugs without the Hot Air. Minimising the Harms of Legal and Illegal Drugs* (Cambridge: UIT 2012).

Pryce, S. *Fixing Drugs. The Politics of Drug Prohibition* (Basingstoke: Palgrave Macmillan, 2012).

Room, R., B. Fischer, W. Hall, S. Lenton, and P. Reuter, *Cannabis Policy. Moving Beyond Stalemate* (Oxford University Press: Beckley Foundation, 2010).

INDEX

alcohol (*cont.*)
  international regulation and 118,
    136–43, 191, 225–7
  medicinal use of 33, 68
  minimum pricing for 3, 226
  new public health approach
    to 190–3, 193
  opium and 18, 24
  prohibition of 48, 49–50, 65, 136,
    139–40, *141*, 142, 144, 190
  regulation of 38, 39, 44–6
  sale of 39, 74–6, 139, 192
  taxation 98, 100–1, 137, 139–40,
    178, 191
  units 96, 233
  urban-rural consumption
    patterns 32–3
  women and 65, 88–95, 140,
    232–7
alcoholism 90
  aversion therapy 223
  'chronic' 68
  disease model of 65, 65–9, 174,
    191, 195
  family studies 89–90
  first use of term 71
  heredity and 64, 89, 90–1
  new 'dependence' term 196, 197
  'problem use' term 199
  substitution treatment of 72;
    see also inebriety
Alford, Bernard 106
alkaloids 7, 29, 30, 69, 97, 108, 109,
  115, 125, 133
alkyl nitrates 2
Allbutt, T. Clifford 71, 113
Alston, Sir Beilby 124, 125, 126
American Association for the Study
  and Cure of Inebriety 62
amphetamines 2, 200

anabolic steroids 2
anaesthetics 9, 115, 116
Anslinger, Harry 227
Anstie, Dr Francis 27, 112–13
anti-opium movement 51–3, 81, 82,
  83, 108, 123, 223
Anti-Saloon League (ASL) 49, 50
anti-slavery movement 37, 43, 121
anti-smoking campaigns 53, 150,
  171–7, 179, 209, 223, 225, 238;
  see also ASH
Arderne, John 9
Argentina 106
Armitage, William 19
Armstrong, Elizabeth M. 235
Armstrong Jones, Sir Ronald 71
Arsenic Acts (1851, 1868) 57
ASBOs (anti-social behaviour
  orders) 236
ASH (Action on Smoking and
  Health) 174–7, 179, 223, 225,
  238
Asia Pacific war (1931-45) 133
ASL (Anti-Saloon League) 48, 49
Asquith, Katherine 160
Asquith, Raymond 160
ATC (American Tobacco
  Company) 105–6
Australia 66, 82, 105, 186–8, 219,
  225, 236
aversion therapy 209, 223

babies 181–3, 184; *see also* children
Bacon, Francis 163
Baddeley, Hermione 162
Bamford, Samuel 32
Band of Hope (temperance
  group) 42
barbiturates 2
Barron, Kevin 237

Royal Commission on Opium report
(1895) 26, 52, 122, 126
Rubinstein, William 102
Rush, Benjamin 66, 67
Russell, Michael 197–9, 206
Russell Smith, Enid 174
Russia 5, 140, 223, 246
Rynd, Dr Francis 111

Saatchi brothers 173–4, 184
Sale of Beer Act (1830) 39
sanitation 73, 120, 167
Scandinavia 71
Scharlieb, Mary 93
Schrad, M. L. 141
science 6, 8, 63, 99, 121, 166–72,
177, 180–2
Scotland 41, 50, 99, 103, 194, 229, 233
seamens' lodging houses 83–4
Second World War (1939-45) 145,
150, 152, 165–7
Seguin, Armand 108
self-help books 18
Serturner, Frederick William 108–9
servicemen 139, 156, 190
Shaftesbury, Lord 51, 61
Shakespeare, William, *Othello* 9–10
Shanghai Protocol (1909) 124–5,
137, 228
Sharkey, Dr Seymour 70
Sherlock Holmes stories 79, 94
Sherwell, Arthur 47, 101
Shipman, Dr Harold 218
Shulgin, Alexander 219
Siam 130, 229
Simon, Sir John 20, 74
Simpson, David 225
Sims, G. R. 79, 93
Single Convention on Narcotic
Drugs (1961) 215

slave trade 137
Smith, George 99
Smith, Professor Goldwin 82
smoking bans 3, 5, 172, 181, 184,
185, 236–8; *see also* cigarettes/
cigarette smoking
smuggling 125, 126, 128, 129, 133,
134, 140, 141, 232
Snowden, C. 203
snuff 9, 33, 34, 74–5, 144, 148;
see also tobacco
social medicine 168, 169, 171–3
social movements 8, 22–3, 36–53,
121, 165, 223–5
anti-opium 50–3, 81, 82, 83, 108,
123, 223
new 174–7, 179, 223, 225, 238;
see also ASH; temperance
movement
Society for the Study and Cure of
Inebriety 60–2, 67–8
Society for the Study of Inebriety
(SSI) 70, 73, 92–3,
126, 167
Society for the Suppression of the
Opium Trade (SSOT) 51–3
sodium bromide 73
solvents 1, 2
Somalia/Somalis 11, 241, 242
Somerset, Lady Henry 44, 49
South Africa 66, 230, 231
Spearman, J. W. 143
spirits 99, 100, 139, 140, 142
Squire, Peter 30
statins 208
Stiles, Thomas 21
strychnine 109
Sturge, Mary 90
Subutex 208
Sun, the 173

Willard, Frances 49
Willcox, Sir William 132
Williams, Sarah 59
Wills, Harry 104
Wilson, Des 175
Wilson, Havelock 82
wine 8, 9, 11, 32, 36, 37, 39, 40, 67,
    96, 100, 140, 142, 157, 178
Wishart, Michael 162
women:
  alcohol and 66, 88–95, 140,
    232–7
  anti-opium campaigns 52
  binge drinking 233, 234
  changing role in society 93–4
  cigarette smoking 143, 145, 148,
    150–2, 152, 154, 181–5, 203
  'doping' children with opiates
    22–3, 167
  drug use 143–5
  'fear' role 78, 232–7, 246
  film stars 148
  'future of the race' and 64, 89, 92,
    94–5, 168, 182, 246
  opium smoking 77, 83, 87–8
  single mothers 183–5
  Somali 241

  in temperance movements 44, 48
Women's Christian Temperance
    Union (WCTU) 49, 142
Wood, C. W. 82–3
Wood, Dr Alexander 111–12
Wood, Mrs Henry, *Danesbury
    House* 40
working class:
  opiates for children 22–3, 167
  opium use 26–7, 57
  political support 46
  smokers 183, 203
  temperance movement and 38,
    41, 42, 44, 48, 50
  women 183–5
workplace smoking bans
    184
World Bank 230
World Health Organization, *see*
    WHO (World Health
    Organization)
Wright, Dr Hamilton 125

Yach, Derek 230, 231
Yeats, W. B. 154, 155
Yemen 241
Yettram, Britannia 158–61